Clinical Manual of Total Cardiovascular Risk

T0075654

Neil R Poulter

Clinical Manual of Total Cardiovascular Risk

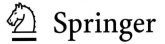 Springer

Neil R Poulter, MBBS, MSc, FRCP
International Centre for Circulatory Health
National Heart and Lung Institute
Imperial College London
London
UK

ISBN 978-1-84800-252-4   e-ISBN 978-1-84800-253-1
DOI 10.1007/978-1-84800-253-1

British Library Cataloguing in Publication Data
A catalogue record for this book is available from the British Library

Library of Congress Control Number: 2008934032

© Springer-Verlag London Limited 2009
Apart from any fair dealing for the purposes of research or private study, or criticism or review, as permitted under the Copyright, Designs and Patents Act 1988, this publication may only be reproduced, stored or transmitted, in any form or by any means, with the prior permission in writing of the publishers, or in the case of reprographic reproduction in accordance with the terms of licences issued by the Copyright Licensing Agency. Enquiries concerning reproduction outside those terms should be sent to the publishers.
The use of registered names, trademarks, etc., in this publication does not imply, even in the absence of a specific statement, that such names are exempt from the relevant laws and regulations and therefore free for general use.
The publisher makes no representation, express or implied, with regard to the accuracy of the information contained in this book and cannot accept any legal responsibility or liability for any errors or omissions that may be made.
Product liability: The publisher can give no guarantee for information about drug dosage and application thereof contained in this book. In every individual case the respective user must check its accuracy by consulting other pharmaceutical literature.

Printed on acid-free paper

Springer Science+Business Media
springer.com

Preface

Over the last 10–20 years, there has been an increasing appreciation of the need to manage individual risk factors for cardiovascular disease (CVD) in the context of overall cv risk rather than on the basis of the absolute level of any given risk factor.

This approach has given rise to the misnomer "global risk" and generated extensive "lip-service" around this more broad-minded approach to managing risk factors and the prevention of CVD.

This short book was devised with the idea of providing a practical summary of the rationale for management based on estimated total CV risk and the various methods associated with so-doing.

Practical issues are addressed including treatment thresholds and targets for the major risk factors on which we routinely intervene, and a brief description of the major means of these interventions is provided.

Whilst a multifactorial approach to CV prevention is logical and reflects the pathophysiological processes which underpin the formation of atherosclerosis, the evidence base to guide practice using estimated CV risk ("global risk") as a threshold for intervention is essentially non-existent.

Meanwhile, pending supportive evidence from randomized trials, practical, pragmatic, and cost-effective approaches to preventing CVD, which is the current biggest contributor to global mortality and burden of disease, is urgently required.

The hope is that this book may make a small contribution toward reducing the horrendous burden which CVD currently imposes on the world.

Contents

Author Biography

Neil R. Poulter, MBBS, MSc, FRCP, is Professor of Preventive Cardiovascular Medicine and Co-Director of the International Centre for Circulatory Health, Imperial College, London, UK. He was President of the British Hypertension Society (BHS) from 2003 to 2005, and was co-author of the 1998 and 2005 Joint British Recommendations on the Prevention of CHD and CVD; the 2003 World Health Organisation/International Society of Hypertension Statement on Management of Hypertension; the 2003 European Society of Hypertension–European Society of Cardiology guidelines for the management of arterial hypertension; and the 2004 BHS guidelines for management of hypertension. He was Director of Operations of the UK half of the ASCOT Trial, and regional Principal Investigator of the North European region of the ADVANCE study. Other Current research interests include the optimal investigation and management of essential hypertension and dyslipidemia, the association between birth weight and hypertension, the cardiovascular effects of exogenous estrogen and progesterone, and ethnic differences in cardiovascular disease and the prevention of type 2 diabetes.

Abbreviations

ABCD-HT	Appropriate Blood Pressure Control in Diabetes hypertensive cohort
ABCD-NT	Appropriate Blood Pressure Control in Diabetes normotensive cohort
ACCOMPLISH	
ACCORD	Action to Control Cardiovascular Risk in Diabetes
ACE	angiotensin-converting enzyme
ADVANCE	Action in Diabetes and Vascular disease: preterAx and diamicroN modified release Controlled Evaluation
ALLHAT	Antihypertensive and Lipid-Lowering treatment to prevent Heart Attack Trial
AMI	acute myocardial infarction
ApoA	apolipoprotein A
ApoB	apolipoprotein B
ARB	angiotensin receptor blocker
ASCOT	Anglo-Scandinavian Cardiac Outcomes Trial
ASCOT-BPLA	Anglo-Scandinavian Cardiac Outcomes Trial–Blood Pressure-Lowering Arm
ASCOT-LLA	Anglo-Scandinavian Cardiac Outcomes Trial–Lipid-Lowering Arm
ATP	Adult Treatment Panel
BHS	British Hypertension Society
BMI	body mass index
BP	blood pressure
BPLTT	Blood Pressure Lowering Treatment Trialists
CARDS	Collaborative AtoRvastatin Diabetes Study
CARE	Cholesterol And Recurrent Events
CCB	calcium-channel blocker
CHD	coronary heart disease
CTT	Cholesterol Treatment Trialists
CV	cardiovascular
CVD	cardiovascular disease
DASH	Dietary Approaches to Stop Hypertension
DBP	diastolic blood pressure
DCCT	Diabetes Control and Complications Trial
DHA	docosahexenoic acid
DIGAMI	Diabetes and Insulin-Glucose infusion in Acute Myocardial Infarction
ECG	electrocardiogram
EPA	eicosapentenoic acid

ESH–ESC	European Society of Hypertension–European Society of Cardiology
EUROPA	EURopean trial On reduction of cardiac events with Perindopril in stable coronary Artery disease
FCH	familial combined hyperlipidemia
FH	familial hypercholesterolemia
GREACE	GREek Atorvastatin and Coronary-heart-disease Evaluation
HbA1c	hemoglobin A1c
HDL	high-density lipoprotein
HMG-CoA	3-Hydroxy-3-methylglutaryl coenzyme A
HOPE	Heart Outcomes Prevention Evaluation
HOT	Hypertension Optimal Treatment
HPS	Heart Protection Study
IDEAL	Incremental Decrease in End points through Aggressive Lipid Lowering
IHD	Ischoemic heart disease
ITT	intention-to-treat
JBS	Joint British Societies
JNC	Joint National Committee on Prevention, Detection, Evaluation, and Treatment of High Blood Pressure
LDL	low-density lipoprotein
LIPID	Long-term Intervention with Pravastatin in Ischemic Disease
LVH	left ventricular hypertrophy
MI	myocardial infarction
MIRACL	Myocardial Ischemia Reduction with Aggressive Cholesterol Lowering
MRFIT	Multiple Risk Factor Intervention Trial
NCEP	National Cholesterol Education Program
NICE	National Institute for Health and Clinical Excellence
NNT	numbers-needed-to-treat
PAR	population attributable risk
PROGRESS	Perindopril pROtection aGainst REcurrent Stroke Study
PROVE-IT	PRavastatin Or atorVastatin Evaluation and Infection Trial
REVERSAL	Reversing Atherosclerosis with Aggressive Lipid Lowering
RCT	randomized controlled trial
SBP	systolic blood pressure
SCORE	Systematic COronary Risk Evaluation
SEARCH	Study of the Effectiveness of Additional Reductions in Cholesterol and Homocysteine
SFA	saturated fatty acid
SHEP	Systolic Hypertension in the Elderly Program
TC	Total Chesterol
TNT	Treating to New Targets
UKPDS	UK Prospective Diabetes Study
WHO–ISH	World Health Organisation–International Society of Hypertension

Chapter 1

Principles of Total Risk Management

Why Assess Total Risk?

Cardiovascular disease (CVD) is a major cause of morbidity and mortality in Western industrialized countries. In the UK, for example, CVD accounted for about 37% of all deaths in 2004. The management of non-fatal stroke and heart attack consumes a major proportion of current healthcare budgets and has a huge detrimental impact on quality of life for both patients and their relatives.

Epidemiological studies indicate that many factors impact on the likelihood of an individual suffering a cardiovascular (CV) event including age, smoking, elevated blood pressure (BP), and cholesterol. The multifactorial nature of CVD and the interactions between risk factors mean that it is difficult for clinicians to make an intuitive assessment of an individual's future risk of disease. This has led to the production of a number of guidelines on the prevention of CVD, all of which recommend risk assessment tools to guide primary prevention strategies.

Individual Risk Factors

The etiology of coronary heart disease (CHD) and stroke has been known for decades to be multifactorial. An increasing risk of both CHD and stroke has been shown to have a graded continuous relationship with rising BP and total cholesterol across the whole BP and cholesterol ranges. Furthermore, among the hypertensive population, for example, the coexistence of other risk factors such as age, smoking, and cholesterol has been shown to result in a dramatic increase in risk associated with any BP stratum. Similarly, among dyslipidemic or diabetic populations, other risk factors have a critical impact on the absolute levels of CV risk for any level of cholesterol or blood glucose.

Significantly, these risk factors tend to cluster in individuals such that, for example, the majority of people with hypertension have at least two other risk factors, and these risk factors are often more common in those with hypertension than in people with a normal BP (see Table 1.1). This clustering

N.R. Poulter, *Clinical Manual of Total Cardiovascular Risk*,
DOI 10.1007/978-1-84800-253-1_1, ©Springer-Verlag London Limited 2009

Table 1.1 Prevalence of other cardiovascular disease risk factors by BP level and sex

Risk factors	Total (%)	
	High BP	Normal BP
Men		
Alcohol >21 units/week	28	30
Cigarette smoker	20	28
Physically inactive	69	46
BMI >25 kg/m2	77	54
Cholesterol >6.5 mmol/l	43	25
Women		
Alcohol >14 units/week	10	15
Cigarette smoker	18	27
Physically inactive	78	56
BMI >25 kg/m2	66	43
Cholesterol >6.5 mmol/l	60	24

BMI, body mass index; BP, blood pressure. Reproduced with permission from Poulter NR et al. *Blood Press* 1996; 5:209–215.

of risk factors is particularly important because, when risk factors coexist, they tend to "interact" such that their combined adverse effect is not only greater than the sum of the individual components (additive), but is usually multiplicative or more (see Fig. 1.1). For example, while the impact of elevated cholesterol on CHD risk appears to be independent of any combination of other risk factors, it is also clear from Table 1.2 that smokers in the highest quintile for serum cholesterol and BP have a risk that is five times greater than non-smokers who have cholesterol in the highest quintile but have a BP in the lowest quintile.

The importance of the interplay of risk factors in determining CHD outcomes was also clearly demonstrated in the results shown in Fig. 1.2. These data show that BP is the most significant predictor of risk in patients with other risk factors.

Consequently, the absolute risk of a CV event occurring in an individual with an elevated level of any given risk factor varies dramatically, perhaps more than 20-fold, depending on the levels of other major determinants of a CV event. It is, therefore, critical not to deal with risk factors in isolation but rather to evaluate a patient's total CV risk and target preventative strategies on that basis. Preventative strategies that do not incorporate some method of risk assessment to guide practice are likely to be less cost-effective. It is important

Fig. 1.1 The multiplicative effect of individual components of risk

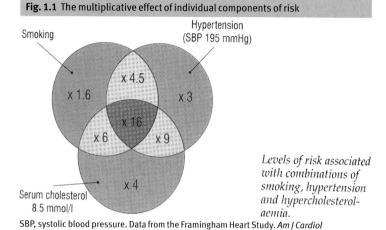

Levels of risk associated with combinations of smoking, hypertension and hypercholesterolaemia.

SBP, systolic blood pressure. Data from the Framingham Heart Study. *Am J Cardiol* 1976; 38:46–51.

to define the frequently misused term "risk factor". Over 250 "risk factors" have been reported in medical journals, many of which do not really cause CHD but have been found, often in isolated studies, to be statistically associated with it. These include "odd" risk factors such as:

- snoring;
- not having siestas;
- non-English mother tongue;
- slow beard growth;
- no varsity athletics at college; and
- poor church attendance.

Deciding which of these statistical associates really do cause CHD and merit the label "risk factor" is subjective and hence a matter of judgment. The recommended criteria whereby an association is judged to be causal usually require a positive response as to whether the association is:

- strong?
- dose-responsive?
- independent?
- consistent?
- apparent with appropriate temporal sequence?
- mechanistically plausible and coherent?
- predictive?
- reversible?

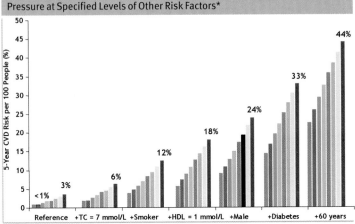

Fig. 1.2 Absolute Risk of CVD over 5 Years in Patients by Systolic Blood Pressure at Specified Levels of Other Risk Factors*

CVD = cardiovascular disease; TC = total cholesterol.
*Risks are given for systolic BP levels from left to right: 110, 120, 130, 140, 150, 160, 170, 180 mm Hg Jackson R et al. *Lancet.* 2005; 365:434–441.

Table 1.3 lists some risk factors that satisfy most of these criteria. It is important to note that, although almost all of these risk factors also increase the risk of stroke, their relative importance is very different for CHD and stroke.

Although CHD and stroke tend to be classified together as the major forms of CVD, their relative incidence rates are very different worldwide (see Table 1.4). This clearly implies that either different levels of the same etiological agents or different agents are at work around the world.

Data, such as those which emerged from the large prospective study of men screened for the Multiple Risk Factor Intervention Trial (MRFIT) (see Table 1.2), demonstrate that the major risk factors for CHD do appear to have been identified, even if their exact role requires fine-tuning.

After 6 years of follow-up, those men screened for MRFIT, who at base-line satisfied all five of the criteria listed below, had a CHD event rate lower than that experienced by Japanese men of the same age who have amongst the lowest CHD death rates in the world:

- non-diabetic;
- non-smokers;
- no previous history of acute myocardial infarction (AMI);
- in the lowest quintile of serum cholesterol; and
- in the lowest quintile of systolic blood pressure (SBP) and diastolic blood pressure (DBP).

Table 1.2 Baseline cigarette smoking, quintiles of serum cholesterol, systolic pressure and age-adjusted CHD mortality per 10,000 person-years

Serum TC	Systolic pressure (mmHg)					Q5/Q1
	<118	118–124	125–131	132–141	142+	
Non smokers						
<182	3.09	3.72	5.13	5.35	13.66	4.42
182–202	4.39	5.79	8.35	7.66	15.8	3.60
203–220	5.20	6.08	8.56	10.72	17.75	3.41
221–244	6.34	9.37	8.66	12.21	22.69	3.58
245+	12.36	12.68	16.31	20.68	33.40	2.70
Q5/Q1	4.00	3.41	3.18	3.87	2.45	–
Smokers						
<182	10.37	10.69	13.21	13.21	27.04	2.61
182–202	10.03	11.76	19.05	20.67	33.69	3.36
203–220	14.90	16.09	21.07	28.87	42.91	2.88
221–244	19.83	22.69	23.61	31.98	55.50	2.80
245+	25.24	30.50	35.26	41.47	62.11	2.46
Q5/Q1	2.43	2.85	2.67	2.96	2.30	

CHD, coronary heart disease; TC, total cholesterol. Q5 is quintile 5; Q1 is quintile 1. Mean follow-up is 11.6 years. (342,815 men free of heart attack and diabetes at baseline were screened for the Multiple Risk Factor Intervention Trial (MRFIT)). Data from Stamler J. Established major coronary risk factors. In: Coronary Heart Disease Epidemiology: From Aetiology to Public Health. Edited by M Marmot, P Elliot. New York: Oxford University Press, 1992; 35–66.

Table 1.3 Risk factors associated with CHD

Modifiable	Non-modifiable
High LDL cholesterol	Age
High BP	Sex
Smoking	Family history
Low HDL cholesterol	
Lack of exercise	
Diabetes (+/– glucose intolerance)	
Left ventricular hypertrophy	
Central obesity	
Clotting factors	
Oral contraceptives	

BP, blood pressure; CHD, coronary heart disease; HDL, high-density lipoprotein; LDL, low-density lipoprotein.

Table 1.4

Number of IHD deaths for each cerebrovascular death

Country	Number of IHD deaths per stroke death
USA	4.63
New Zealand	4.19
Australia	3.61
England & Wales	3.58
Singapore	2.20
Sri Lanka	1.94
France	1.44
Hong Kong	0.91
Japan	0.46
Korea	0.08

IHD, ischemic heart disease

At 10.5 years of follow-up (see Table 1.5), the mortality data of those considered at low risk compared with all those screened at baseline appear to emphasize that the major risk factors for CHD are:

- dyslipidemia;
- smoking;
- raised BP; and
- diabetes.

These data powerfully vindicate the belief that public health policy should be aimed toward improving lipid profiles, stopping smoking, lowering BP, and decreasing obesity. Furthermore, this policy should now be reinforced more strongly.

In 2004, the INTERHEART study—the largest ever case-control study of AMI carried out in almost 30,000 men and women of all ages from 50 countries worldwide—highlighted the fact that the vast majority of the etiological determinants of CHD have been identified and, furthermore, are preventable. In this huge study, nine risk factors explained 90% and 94% of the population attributable risk (PAR) among men and women, respectively (see Fig. 1.3 and Table 1.6).

Importantly, smoking, dyslipidemia (as assessed by the ApoB/ApoA ratio), and hypertension contributed to the majority of the estimated PAR, and three important protective factors—exercise, intake of alcohol, and fresh fruit and vegetables—were clearly identified. Finally, it should be noted that the role of genetics is left to play a minor role (if any at all) in this large, worldwide, population-based study.

Table 1.5 MRFIT screenees: 10.5-year mortality rates/1000*

Cause of death	Low-risk† men	All men
CHD	2.0	17.4
Cancer	11.8	16.4
All causes	23.9	49.3

*Age adjusted. †Non-smoker, non-diabetic, no history of acute myocardial infarction, total cholesterol <4.7 mmol/l, systolic pressure <120 mmHg, diastolic pressure <80 mmHg.

The data arising from the MRFIT and INTERHEART studies suggest that at least for simple everyday risk assessment, few, if any, other major risk factors need to be considered. Nevertheless, much emphasis has been placed on biomarkers and particularly on high-sensitivity C-reactive protein. This fashionable focus relates to beliefs that vascular inflammation may be

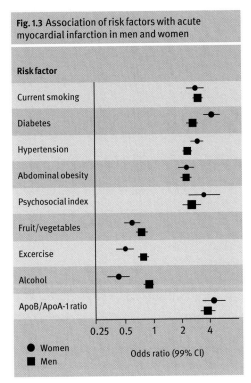

Fig. 1.3 Association of risk factors with acute myocardial infarction in men and women

Risk factor

- Current smoking
- Diabetes
- Hypertension
- Abdominal obesity
- Psychosocial index
- Fruit/vegetables
- Excercise
- Alcohol
- ApoB/ApoA-1 ratio

0.25 0.5 1 2 4

● Women
■ Men

Odds ratio (99% CI)

Apo, alipoprotein; CI, confidence interval. Results were adjusted for age, sex, and geographical region. Reproduced with permission from Yusuf S et al. *Lancet* 2004; 364:937–952.

Table 1.6 Association of risk factors with acute myocardial infarction in men and women after adjustment for age, sex, and geographic region

Risk factor	Sex	Control (%)	Case (%)	Odds ratio (99%CI)	PAR (99% CI)
Current smoking	F	9.3	20.1	2.86 (2.36–3.48)	15.8% (12.9–19.3)
	M	33.0	53.1	3.05 (2.78–3.33)	44.0% (40.9–47.2)
Diabetes	F	7.9	25.5	4.26 (3.51–5.18)	19.1% (16.8–21.7)
	M	7.4	16.2	2.67 (2.36–3.02)	10.1% (8.9–11.4)
Hypertension	F	28.3	53.0	2.95 (2.57–3.39)	35.8% (32.1–39.6)
	M	19.7	34.6	2.32 (2.12–2.53)	19.5% (17.7–21.5)
Abdominal obesity	F	33.3	45.6	2.26 (1.90–2.68)	35.9% (28.9–43.6)
	M	33.3	46.5	2.24 (2.03–2.47)	32.1% (28.0–36.5)
Psychosocial index	F	–	–	3.49 (2.41–5.04)	40.0% (28.6–52.6)
	M	–	–	2.58 (2.11–3.14)	25.3% (18.2–34.0)
Fruit/vegetables	F	50.3	39.4	0.58 (0.48–0.71)	17.8% (12.9–24.1)
	M	39.6	34.7	0.74 (0.66–0.83)	10.3% (6.9–15.2)
Exercise	F	16.5	9.3	0.48 (0.39–0.59)	37.3% (26.1–50.0)
	M	20.3	15.8	0.77 (0.69–0.85)	22.9% (16.9–30.2)
Alcohol	F	11.2	6.3	0.41 (0.32–0.53)	46.9% (34.3–60.0)
	M	29.1	29.6	0.88 (0.81–0.96)	10.5% (6.1–17.5)
ApoB/ApoA ratio	F	14.1	27.0	4.42 (3.43–5.70)	52.1% (44.0–60.2)
	M	21.9	35.5	3.76 (3.23–4.38)	53.8% (48.3–59.2)

CI, confidence interval; PAR, population attributable risk. Reproduced with permission from Yusuf et al. *Lancet* 2004; 364:937–952.

a primary determinant of atherosclerosis rather than an epi-phenomenon associated with raised and/or atherogenic low-density lipoprotein (LDL) cholesterol.

This debate notwithstanding, elevated high-sensitivity C-reactive protein is not a particularly strong risk factor for CVD (see Table 1.7) and, given its lack of specificity and sensitivity for CV events, not to mention the cost of measuring it, its value in terms of risk assessment is, at best, questionable. By contrast, several of the simple, easily measured variables in Table 1.7

Table 1.7 Risk variables for cardiovascular and cerebrovascular disease

Variable	Event	RR
C-reactive protein*	CHD	1.8
Migraine	Ischemic CVA	3.5
Pulse†	CV death	2.0
Creatinine‡	CV death	1.5–2.75

CHD, coronary heart disease; CV, cardiovascular; CVA, cerebrovascular accident.
*>3 mg/l vs <1.0 g/l; †<60 vs <100; ‡Q1 vs Q5.

Table 1.8 Development and standard risk factors

	Rises	Falls
Age	x	
Exercise		x
Alcohol intake	x	
Salt intake	x	
Potassium intake		x
Body weight	x	
Stress	?	
Smoking	x	
Saturated fats	x	

reproduced with permission from poulter NR. Current Issues in Hypertension. Oxford: Bladon Medical Publishimg, 2004.

should probably influence intervention over and above the determination of CV risk using conventional algorithms.

Whatever the composition of a list of "favorite" risk factors for CVD, it is clear that the key determinants of the "major" risk factors—dyslipidemia, hypertension, smoking, and diabetes—are attributable to a "Westernized" lifestyle.

Table 1.8 shows the impact of development on standard risk factors and highlights the pivotal role of the environment in determining CV events throughout the world. By implication, the positive take on these data is that most CV events are preventable.

Chapter 2

Identifying the Patient at Risk

Total Risk—Methods of Assessment

Realization that CV risk could not be accurately assessed on the basis of data for a single risk factor (e.g., being dyslipidemic or not) has been acknowledged for over 20 years. However, as recently as 1991, medical algorithms for risk factor management were described as "while paying lip-service to the others, consider them one at a time."

Published Guidelines

The 1993 British Hypertension Society (BHS) guidelines mentioned coexisting risk factors as possible determinants of lowering BP treatment thresholds, but these recommendations were not specific, defined, or qualified, and consequently were not incorporated into routine clinical practice in any systematic way. The belief that experienced clinicians could judge risk status without a formal tool to do so was not supported by a French study in which six hypertension specialists were asked to assign 100 patients to low-, moderate-, or high-risk categories. The proportions of patients assigned to each category ranged from 23% to 77% for the low-risk and from 4.5% to 44% for the high-risk groups.

The Joint National Committee on Prevention, Detection, Evaluation, and Treatment of High Blood Pressure (JNC 6) guidelines from the USA introduced a crude risk classification method to guide treatment thresholds. These guidelines recommended that patients be classified into one of three categories of coexistent risk factors (from nil to established disease or target organ damage) for each of three or four grades of BP. One study attempted to validate this approach by calculating the numbers needed to treat (NNT) to prevent one CV event or one death by lowering SBP by 12 mmHg in each stratum. In essence, the results of this study confirmed that, despite its crude nature, this approach did differentiate those at highest risk from those at a lower risk. This type of risk stratification was subsequently adopted by the World Health Organisation–International

N.R. Poulter, *Clinical Manual of Total Cardiovascular Risk*,
DOI 10.1007/978-1-84800-253-1_2, Springer-Verlag London Limited 2009

Society of Hypertension (WHO–ISH) guidelines produced in 1999 and in their follow-up statement in 2003.

Several other more complex and more accurate methods of predicting relatively short-term risk of either a CHD event or a CV event (stroke or CHD) have been developed. The most commonly used risk scores have arisen from the algorithm derived from the Framingham cohort and in relation to coronary rather than CV risk. Several established risk factors are not included in some of the risk scores, in part because risk charts, for logistical reasons, cannot include more than a few variables and also because the original cohort studies that provided the risk-assessment databases did not measure some of the factors that clearly do impact independently on risk.

The exclusion of risk factors such as pulse rate, microalbuminuria, exercise, and migraine inevitably means that at the individual level, risk scores may be significantly inaccurate. Furthermore, the risk associated with some of the risk factors may be miscalculated, usually because some of the risk factors, such as smoking or diabetes, are treated dichotomously—either present or absent. The result is inaccuracy and misclassification, because it is clear in the case of diabetes, for example, that the risk associated with glycemia, as assessed by HbA1c level, is graded and continuous and the level of risk is further affected by duration of the diagnosis. Similarly, regarding smoking-related risk, a person who has smoked one cigarette per day for the last 2 years may be classified as a smoker, whereas someone who stopped smoking 5 years ago, having smoked 60 cigarettes per day for 30 years, may be considered a non-smoker. Such classification will inevitably produce inaccurate results.

Despite the shortcomings of the Framingham database—which was based on a relatively small, mainly white, middle-class cohort from Massachusetts—the score it produces has been shown to be reasonably accurate when applied to the northern European setting. Its generalizability to southern Europe and other ethnic subgroups, however, is less clear.

Whatever the setting, it appears that the Framingham risk score ranks people well in terms of CV risk, although the absolute levels of risk across the rankings may be seriously inaccurate. However, using relatively limited local data, the score can be reset to adjust for background site-specific conditions and the score can then not only rank risk effectively, but is also accurate for absolute risk prediction. Results such as these mean that in situations where finances or the infrastructure to carry out site-specific, large-scale epidemiological cohort studies (necessary to generate accurate local risk scores) are unavailable, statistical manipulation of the Framingham risk score supported by relatively limited local data can generate useful locally accurate risk charts.

Nevertheless, early European guidelines produced a chart based on the Framingham algorithm to help evaluate the risk of developing CHD. These charts were improved upon by including high-density lipoprotein (HDL) cholesterol and incorporated into the New Zealand charts, which could be used to estimate the 5-year risk of a CV event.

These charts were refined and simplified, and incorporated into the 1998 Joint British Societies (JBS) guidelines (produced jointly by the British Cardiac Society, British Hyperlipidaemic Association, and British Hypertension Society [BHS], and endorsed by the British Diabetic Association), although this group, for reasons of consistency with European and Scottish guidelines, reverted to evaluating coronary risk. This chart, like all others of its kind, has one consistent and important inherent problem—it only predicts short-term (usually 5 or 10 years) absolute risk, which is used as a key determinant of intervention. This causes under-treatment of young people at high relative risk and over-treatment of older people at lower relative risk. For example, a 32-year-old woman, even if she is diabetic, a smoker, has a total cholesterol to HDL ratio of 8 and an SBP of 170 mmHg, does not reach the 10-year 30% risk of CHD threshold—the level at which intervention was recommended. In contrast, most elderly men would qualify for intervention simply on account of their age and sex. The European approach to offset this problem was to "project" young people with high levels of risk factors to age 60 and to base treatment decisions on the resulting estimated level of risk. This is one way of reducing the ageism and sexism inherent in current risk-assessment charts.

The 1998 JBS guidelines produced a user-friendly computerized risk assessor, which included a larger number of variables than in their chart and so provided a more accurate risk calculation for both CHD and stroke. However, of the nine variables included in the risk assessor, three of them—smoking, diabetes, and left ventricular hypertrophy (LVH) on ECG—are dealt with dichotomously, with all the shortcomings of such an approach as described above.

It should be noted that the Framingham risk equation, which underpins all of these charts, relates not only to fatal CHD and non-fatal myocardial infarction (MI), but also to silent MI and "coronary insufficiency"—presumably equivalent to unstable angina. Conscious of criticism that this score over-predicted risk in certain situations, a new score was produced in the third Adult Treatment Panel (ATP III) report from the National Cholesterol Education Program (NCEP), based on "harder" endpoints—fatal CHD and stroke, and non-fatal MI and stroke.

In clinical practice, however, both the prescribing doctor and the patient are likely to be interested in all major CV events (including stroke and heart failure) and procedures such as angioplasty and bypass grafting, rather than just fatal and non-fatal CHD, and certainly not just fatal events. In 2004 the JBS upgraded their tables, published initially as part of the 2004 BHS guidelines and subsequently in the JBS 2 guidelines (see Fig. 2.1). These tables differed from and improved upon those included in the simplified 1998 JBS guidelines in the following ways:

- CV risk (fatal and non-fatal MI and stroke) was considered and not just CHD risk;
- only three age strata were included (<50, 50–59, and >60 years). These three strata are actually calculated for 49, 59, and 69 year olds respectively. By so doing, some of the concerns of not treating young people at high relative but low absolute short-term risk are reduced. Similarly, the propensity to treat everyone over the age of 75 based on short-term absolute risk is tempered; and
- no charts for patients with diabetes are included because, with the exception of a very small subgroup of the youngest and female patients, the estimated CV risk is always >20% over 10 years (i.e., in the red area in Fig. 2.1).

The value of using an approach to BP management based on CV risk rather than a BP threshold has been evaluated in one study which confirmed that, depending on the threshold used, fewer people could be treated and more events prevented by the risk-based approach.

More recently, the INDIANA project has produced a risk score that used the results of eight randomized controlled trials (RCTs) of hypertension management as the database. This method generated a score based on 11 variables that predict CV death. This is the first score to incorporate serum creatinine and height as determinants of risk, but also includes established history of MI and stroke. Given that most management guidelines do not use risk assessment for those with established disease because treatment is supplied to all such people anyway, the value of the score is limited.

A more recent risk score produced in Europe is the one that has emerged from the SCORE project. Based on 12 European cohort studies—mainly population-based studies, including about 2.7 million years of follow-up—a chart or computer-based system of predicting stroke or CHD death ("CV death") was developed.

Acknowledging the important impact of differences on background rates of CV death, risk estimation charts have been produced for high and low CV

Fig. 2.1 Joint British Societies" cardiovascular disease risk: non-diabetic population

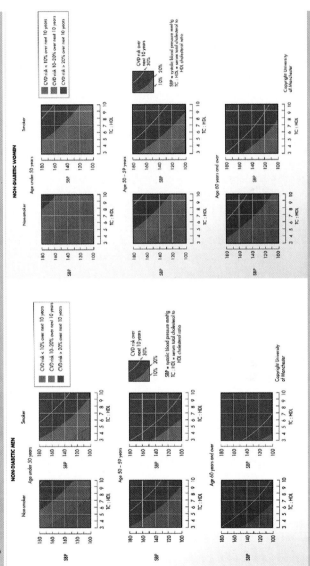

BP, blood pressure; CVD, cardiovascular disease; HDL, high-density lipoprotein; TC, total cholesterol. Reproduced with permission from the JBS 2 guidelines. *Heart* 2005; 91(Suppl 5):1–52.

event populations, with or without the inclusion of HDL cholesterol. The latter modification reflects major differences of opinion within Europe regarding the importance of HDL cholesterol in risk calculation, not to mention its availability as a routine measure. The authors of the SCORE project report no effect of the inclusion or exclusion of HDL in their risk-prediction model, while counter arguments propose that this reflects different and inadequate measurements of HDL in the various studies that form the database. An additional advantage of the computerized version of the SCORE system is the ability to incorporate whatever additional "favorite" risk factor the user may wish as an extra dimension.

Clearly, the major downside to this system, as discussed above, is that the outcome measure—CV death—is not the one patients and doctors are most concerned about. Furthermore, the charts are complicated (see Fig. 2.2) and incorporate a new range of numbers that doctors (who are only just getting to grips with 10-year CHD or CV risk thresholds of 15%, 20% or 30%) are likely to find confusing.

A further problem with the SCORE system is that diabetic subjects were included at baseline in the databases of the cohorts used, and results cannot be differentiated for diabetic and non-diabetic subjects. The recommendation for calculating risk in diabetic subjects using this method, therefore, is to double the estimate calculated for males and quadruple that estimated for females. This is clearly crude and probably provides little, if anything, over Framingham-based calculations with their well-established limitations due to small numbers.

In summary, therefore, all risk-assessment tools, by virtue of limited and misclassified variables, are inevitably inaccurate and should only provide guidance in the context of all the available information gleaned from a thorough medical investigation. The ideal requirements of a risk factor-scoring system are summarized in Table 2.1. What is clear is that many of these requirements contradict each other. For example, to be valid, a score needs to be comprehensive, which pre-empts the requirements of simplicity, being cheap and user-friendly.

Nevertheless, the assessment of total CV risk (frequently misnamed "global" risk) is increasingly endorsed and encouraged as a guide to clinical practice, and strategies that do not incorporate such an approach are likely to be less cost-effective and/or affordable.

The trade-off between accuracy and simplicity can only be ultimately realized by computerized systems, which incorporate many more variables. This assumes that data on all these variables are likely to become routinely collected. Meanwhile, the ideal system should predict major CV (rather than coronary)

Fig. 2.2 Ten-year risk of fatal CVD in high-risk regions of Europe by gender, age, SBP, total cholesterol and smoking status

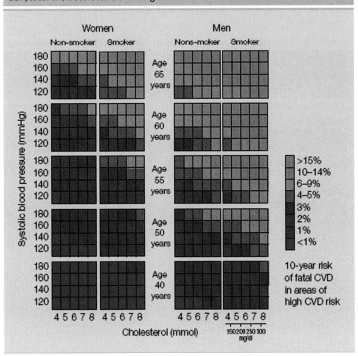

CVD, cardiovascular disease; SBP, systolic blood pressure. Reproduced with permission from Conroy RM et al. *Eur Heart J* 2003; 24:987–1003.

events (fatal and non-fatal) and incorporate some method of avoiding the shortcomings of predicting only short-term absolute risk. To date, admittedly with more emphasis on simplicity than accuracy, the charts produced in the BHS IV and the JBS 2 guidelines of 2005 are the best available option. This tool, like all of the others available, should be used to guide rather than rule the practice by clinicians who should be fully aware of the shortcomings of the system in use. These latest BHS guidelines provide a simple clear summary of what (and who) should be screened to allow effective risk assessment:

- all adults aged 40 and above, who have no history of CVD or diabetes, and who are not already on treatment for BP or lipids; and
- younger adults (<40 years) with a family history of premature athero-sclerotic disease.

Table 2.1 Risk factor scoring system – ideal requirements

1 Simple

2 Comprehensive

3 Cheap

4 Valid (predictive)

5 User friendly

6 Easily interpreted by
  – doctor
  – patient

7 Useful to
  – identify
  – motivate
  – monitor
  – improve management

Risk assessment should include ethnicity, smoking habit history, family history of CVD, and measurements of weight, waist circumference, BP, non-fasting lipids (total cholesterol and HDL cholesterol), and non-fasting glucose. CVD risk prediction charts from JBS 2 (see Fig. 2.1) should be used to estimate total risk of developing CVD (CHD and stroke) over 10 years based on five risk factors: age, sex, smoking habit, SBP, and the ratio of total cholesterol to HDL cholesterol. This is the estimated probability (percentage chance) of developing CVD over the next 10 years and is referred to as total CVD risk. Total CVD risk should be estimated for the person's current age group: <50 years, 50–59 years, or ≥60 years. A total CVD risk of >20% over 10 years is defined as "high risk" and requires professional lifestyle intervention and, where appropriate, drug therapies to achieve the lifestyle and risk factor targets.

When assessing and managing a person's overall CVD risk, other risk factors not included in the CVD risk prediction charts should be taken into account, including:

• ethnic group—in people originating from the Indian subcontinent it is reasonable to assume that CVD risk is about 1.4 times higher than predicted from the charts;

• abdominal obesity (waist circumference: men >102 cm, women >88 cm, and in Asians >90 cm in men and >80 cm in women) increases the risk of diabetes and CVD;

- impaired glucose regulation is defined as impaired fasting glucose (IFG) or impaired glucose tolerance (IGT), and both are associated with an increased risk of developing diabetes and CVD. If non-fasting glucose is ⩾6.1 mmol/l, then fasting glucose should be measured for evidence of impaired glucose regulation or new diabetes;
- raised fasting triglyceride (>1.7 mmol/l) increases the risk of CVD; and
- a family history of premature CVD, and especially CHD (men <55 years and women <65 years) in a first-degree relative increases the risk of developing CVD by about 1.3.

Risk assessments should be repeated, ideally within 5 years, in those not found to be at high total CVD risk using the comprehensive CV risk assessment based on the JBS charts, or in those started for other reasons on drug therapy to lower BP, lipids, or glucose. Under the age of 40, the 10-year total CVD risk will usually be low, but the risk can be extrapolated to older age groups, assuming risk factors do not change. Over the age of 70, CVD risk is usually ⩾20% over 10 years, especially for men, but total CVD risk should still be formally estimated using the charts, even though this will underestimate the true total CVD risk of a person older than 70 years.

Special Considerations

The Developing World

Cognizant of the fact that in many parts of the world resources do not allow measurement of the limited number of risk factors used in the standard risk-assessment algorithm, WHO have generated a series of risk charts for different geographical areas. The utility of these charts, which were introduced in 2006, remains to be seen.

Established CVD

Risk assessment in those with established CVD—expressed in terms of symptoms of CHD, cerebrovascular or peripheral arterial disease—is largely unnecessary. People in this category are clearly at high risk of developing a further major CV event or of death. Consequently, such patients merit – on the basis of extensive trial evidence – intervention on all the standard risk factors using the whole range of currently available CV protective agents. Further evaluation of risk status may, in a small minority of cases, affect the intensity of interventions applied, but, for the vast majority, risk assessment is of little or no routine value.

Diabetes

The need for risk estimation among diabetic subjects is, in itself, controversial. In the most recent ATP III report the recommendation is to consider those with type 2 diabetes as "coronary equivalents", thereby obviating the need for risk assessment.

This recommendation is based on one Finnish study, which conflicts with other epidemiological data. However, the evidence strongly suggests that the CHD risk among diabetic subjects aged above 50 or those who have been diagnosed for at least 10 years is equivalent to that of post-MI patients. Furthermore, the short- and long-term case fatality rates for patients with diabetes is much higher than for those without. Hence for simplicity, given that most patients with type 2 diabetes are aged over 50, it seems reasonable to treat this group as coronary equivalents, which in turn pre-empts the need for "global risk" estimation. However, a risk scoring system ("engine") has been developed, based on the UK Prospective Diabetes Study (UKPDS) trial, for patients with diabetes. While this is undoubtedly a more accurate tool for assessing diabetic risk than any other method available, its value may be restricted to the small number of patients aged below 50 who have been diabetic for less than 10 years.

Those with IFG ($\geq$6.1 mmol/l but <7.0 mmol/l) or IGT (2-hour plasma glucose $\geq$7.8 mmol/l and <11.1 mmol/l in an oral glucose tolerance test) are at increased risk of developing type 2 diabetes and of developing CVD compared with normoglycemic individuals.

For all practical purposes, those with type 1 diabetes can be considered together with patients with type 2 diabetes.

Obesity and the Metabolic Syndrome

Obesity, hypertension, and diabetes overlap to a considerable extent among communities in which any of the three conditions are prevalent. Clearly, a common etiological thread, such as physical inactivity, may be driving all three problems.

Recent interest has been focused on pre-diabetic conditions, variously described as syndrome X, the insulin-resistance syndrome, or the metabolic syndrome. The value of the latter term has been debated recently and it has been defined in several ways (see Table 2.2). The most recent definition, proposed by the International Diabetes Federation in 2005, appears the most useful and pragmatic by placing central obesity at the core of the "syndrome".

However, the controversial value of the syndrome notwithstanding the metabolic syndrome is essentially a constellation of metabolic and non-metabolic disorders relating to defects in insulin sensitivity that

Table 2.2 Metabolic syndrome definitions

NCEP–ATP III definition

Any three or more of the following criteria:
- Waist circumference ›102 cm in men and ›88 cm in women
- Serum triglycerides ›1.7
- BP ›130/85
- HDL-C ‹1.0 in men and ‹1.3 in women
- Serum glucose ›6.1 (5.6 may be applicable)

WHO definition

Diabetes, IFG, IGT or insulin resistance (clamp studies) and at least two of the following criteria:
- Waist–hip ratio ›0.90 in men or ›0.85 in women
- Serum triglycerides ›1.7 or HDL-C ‹0.9 in men and ‹1.0 in women
- BP ›140/90
- Urinary albumin excretion ›20 µg/min or albumin–creatinine ratio ›30 mg/g

IDF 2005 worldwide metabolic syndrome definition

Central obesity
- Waist circumference ≥94 cm for men and ≥80 cm for women (Europid values)

Plus at least two of the following:
- TG level ≥150 mg/dl (≥1.7 mmol/l) or treatment for hypertriglyceridemia
- HDL-C ‹40 mg/dl (‹1.03 mmol/l) in males and ‹50 mg/dl (‹1.29 mmol/l) in females or treatment for reduced HDL-C
- Systolic BP ≥130 mmHg or diastolic BP ≥85 mmHg or treatment for hypertension
- Fasting plasma glucose ≥100 mg/dl (≥5.6 mmol/l) or type 2 diabetes

BP, blood pressure; HDL-C, high-density lipoprotein cholesterol; IFG, impaired fasting glucose; IGT, impaired glucose tolerance; TG, triglyceride. Data from NCEP Expert Panel. *Circulation* 2002; 106:3143–3421; Alberti KG et al. *Diabet Med* 1998; 15:539–553; Alberti KG et al. *Lancet* 2005; 366:1059–1062.

ultimately lead to an increased risk of developing type 2 diabetes and CVD. In population-based studies in a multi-ethnic community, approximately one-quarter of all adults without diabetes or evidence of CVD at baseline were identified as having the metabolic syndrome using the ATP III guideline definition. In observational studies over a follow-up period of about 10 years, the incidence of CVD events among those with this "syndrome" was found to be approximately twice that of the control population. The presence of the metabolic syndrome, so defined, increases the incidence of subsequent type 2 diabetes by three to fourfold. The greater the number of features of the metabolic syndrome, the greater is the subsequent risk of CVD events, although synergy among the components of the "syndrome" is less clear. Worldwide studies demonstrate that the prevalence of the metabolic syndrome, however defined, is increasing along with accompanying obesity, and hence type 2 diabetes. This means that an increasing number of individuals, as a result of modest increases in a few coexistent risk factors—as in the metabolic syndrome—are at moderate risk of CVD despite having sub-threshold levels for the treatment of any of the individual risk factors.

Other Subgroups

Formal risk assessment of patients with established target organ damage (e.g., LVH, renal damage) as opposed to established vascular disease are not available. Nevertheless, most sets of guidance recommend that these people be classified along with those who have established vascular disease (i.e., being at high CV risk). Hence, they are recommended to receive interventive strategies at lower thresholds than those without target organ damage. In the JBS 2 guidelines of 2005, intervention is recommended on the basis of the status of various single risk factors, independent of total risk assessment. For example, those with an SBP ≥160 mmHg or DBP ≥100 mmHg should receive antihypertensive medication irrespective of total risk. Similarly, it is recommended that those with a total cholesterol to HDL cholesterol ratio ≥6 should receive lipid-lowering therapy irrespective of the total risk status. These recommendations, to some extent, fly in the face of the ideal total risk-assessment approach to management but in part reflect historical practice and the RCT evidence—particularly in the case of hypertension, where drug intervention is also relatively cheap. It should also be appreciated that such recommendations are totally commensurate with the classical treatment policy for "diabetes", whereby dysglycemia is treated as a dichotomous variable that needs intervention at a particular cut-point, independent of any assessment of lipids, BP, or other risk factor.

Chapter 3

Strategies for Cardiovascular Risk Management

Lifestyle Modification

Although the benefits of non-pharmacological measures in terms of pre-venting CV events are by no means established, the lifestyle changes rec-ommended in all recent sets of guidelines for CVD prevention, whether by means of lowering BP, lipids, or glucose, are likely to benefit the whole of society, irrespective of the level of any of the individual risk factors. At the very worst, these changes are deemed harmless. It is a fact, however, that the extensive trial evidence relating to non-drug measures that does exist almost exclusively relates to benefits in terms of improving risk factor levels rather than on the prevention of major CV events.

There is some confusion over the interpretation of the efficacy of such lifestyle interventions. In studies in which compliance with dietary interven-tions is achieved (e.g., reduction of fat intake to lower cholesterol), benefits on risk factors (e.g., blood lipid levels) have clearly been shown, although these studies have mainly been of short duration. However, when compli-ance with dietary measures has not been achieved, no benefits have accrued. Based on the intention-to-treat (ITT) principle, this has been misinterpreted to mean that "diets don't work." A more realistic summary of the situation is that the ability of health professionals to persuade patients to change their diet and lifestyle is limited. However, if and when healthy lifestyles are taken up, there do seem to be benefits, albeit on surrogate endpoints.

Based on evidence from both epidemiology and clinical trials, several lifestyle measures can improve CV risk-factor profiles and reduce the incidence of CV events among asymptomatic people or those with established CVD. Indeed, for many people whose total CVD risk is not sufficiently high to justify pharmacotherapy at their present age, lifestyle intervention can be the only approach offered for CVD prevention. However, where the total risk of CVD is sufficiently high to justify more intensive intervention, or when the level of any one risk factor is already associated with target organ damage, lifestyle measures alone are usually not sufficient and drugs will also be required to

N.R. Poulter, *Clinical Manual of Total Cardiovascular Risk*,
DOI 10.1007/978-1-84800-253-1_3, Springer-Verlag London Limited 2009

Table 3.1 Lifestyle targets

- Do not smoke
- Maintain ideal body weight for adults (BMI 20–25-kg/m2) and avoid central obesity (waist circumference in white Caucasians <102 cm in men and <88 cm in women, and in Asians <90 cm in men and <80 cm in women)
- Keep total dietary intake of fat to <30% of total energy intake
- Keep the intake of saturated fats to <10% of total fat intake
- Keep the intake of dietary cholesterol to <300 mg/day
- Replace saturated fats by an increased intake of monounsaturated fats
- Increase the intake of fresh fruit and vegetables to at least five portions per day
- Regular intake of fish and other sources of omega-3 fatty acids (at least two servings of fish per week)
- Limit alcohol intake to <21 units/week for men or <14 units/week for women
- Limit the intake of salt to <100 mmol/l day (<6 g of sodium chloride or <2.4 g of sodium per day)
- Regular aerobic physical activity of at least 30 minutes per day, most days of the week, should be taken (e.g., fast walking/swimming)

BMI, body mass index. Reproduced with permission from the JBS 2 guidelines. *Heart* 2005; 91(Suppl 5):1–52.

achieve targets. In addition to professional support, the involvement of the patient's partner and all family members living in the same household may be helpful in making lifestyle changes, such as those listed in Table 3.1.

Smoking

Smoking (including passive smoking) increases the risk of CVD in a way that is related to the amount of tobacco smoked daily and the duration of smoking, and the absolute adverse impact of smoking is greater in those with other risk factors such as hypertension or diabetes. In people with CHD, stopping smoking can be followed by a rapid decline in the risk of a further CHD event, by as much as 50% after 1 year, and within 2–3 years the risk falls to the level of those people with CHD who have never smoked. In asymptomatic people, it can take up to 10 years to reach the risk level of those people who have never smoked.

All cigarette smokers should receive advice from a doctor to stop smoking completely and this advice should be reiterated and reinforced by all health professionals. Such advice has proved to be effective and should ideally include:

- description of the CV risks (and other disease risks) of smoking;
- provision of appropriate information on approaches to stopping;
- assessment of readiness to stop; and
- agreeing a specific plan with a follow-up arrangement.

In the initial period of stopping smoking, nicotine replacement therapy (e.g., chewing gum or transdermal patches) can almost double cessation rates. In addition, nicotine patches have been tested in people with coronary disease without any adverse effects. Antidepressant medications in the form of bupropion and nortriptyline can also help, and selective cannabinoid-1 receptor blockers and other therapeutic approaches may have a role in the future.

Diet

There are complex relationships between diet and CVD, but the epidemiological evidence shows that total fat, and specifically saturated fatty acids (SFAs), are both positively associated with coronary mortality. As consumption of SFAs increases, so does LDL cholesterol. Replacing saturated fats with monounsaturated or polyunsaturated fats reduces the risk of CV events and reduces LDL but also reduces HDL or 'good' cholestrol.

Sources of polyunsaturated fatty acids include vegetable oils such as soybean, safflower, and linseed oils. An RCT of a diet enriched with α-linoleic acid in high-risk people has shown reductions in coronary and all-cause mortality. Eicosapentenoic acid (EPA) and docosahexenoic acid (DHA) are principally obtained from fish and some vegetable oils (e.g., soybean oil). Epidemiological studies show regular fish consumers to be at lower risk of fatal CHD, including sudden death. RCTs in people with established coronary disease have shown that increased fish consumption and supplementation of EPA/DHA produce reductions in coronary and total mortality.

Plant stenols or sterols that have been esterified to increase their lipid solubility can be incorporated into food and will reduce the absorption of cholesterol from the gut and lower blood cholesterol values. Adding 2 g of plant stenol or sterol to an average portion of margarine reduces LDL cholesterol by an average of about 0.5 mmol/l in middle-aged people, which would be expected to reduce the risk of CHD by about 25% over 2 years.

Trans-fatty acids are usually derived from industrial hydrogenation of mono-unsaturated or polyunsaturated fats and in some epidemiological studies dietary intake is positively related to the risk of CVD. Dietary cholesterol has relatively little effect on blood lipid values, but in metabolic studies there is considerable variation in response between individuals, and dietary cholesterol intake has been related to the development of CHD in some epidemiological studies.

In epidemiological studies, fruit and vegetable consumption has been found to be inversely related to CHD risk but, apart from one trial in hypertension, there is no other RCT evidence. In the DASH (Dietary Approaches to Stop Hypertension) trial, a diet rich in fruit, vegetables, and low-fat dairy products with reduced content of both total and saturated fat was found to reduce BP. Reduced sodium intake, especially in the form of sodium chloride, will also reduce BP. RCTs of vitamin supplementation have failed to demonstrate any benefit on CVD mortality or total mortality.

Alcohol

Alcohol consumption of 1–3 units of alcohol per day (a unit equates to about 80 ml of wine, 250 ml of normal strength beer, and 30–50 ml of spirits) is associated with lower coronary mortality. Optimum consumption is lower for women than men. There is no evidence of any difference in CV benefit of any one source of alcohol compared with another. The pattern of alcohol use also has an effect on CV risk; binge drinking (i.e., consuming five or more drinks at a time) is associated with a higher risk of sudden death and stroke. There is an increased risk of hemorrhagic stroke and, to a lesser extent, ischemic stroke above 3 units per day. As alcohol consumption increases above 3 units per day, so does SBP and DBP, the risk of cardiac arrhythmias, cardiomyopathy, and sudden death.

Physical Activity

Physical activity, either at work or in leisure time, is associated with a lower risk of CHD in both men and women, and has a beneficial effect on other CV risk factors. It helps to promote losing weight and to prevent weight gain. Physical activity can prevent or delay the development of high BP, increases HDL cholesterol concentration, and reduces the risk of developing diabetes.

In asymptomatic people, aerobic physical activity and cardiorespiratory fitness are associated with a significant reduction in CV and all-cause mortality. The largest reduction in risk is between sedentary and moderately active individuals, with a more modest reduction between moderate and vigorous activity. This CV benefit is lost when physical activity is discontinued. In people with established CHD the most recent meta-analysis of RCTs of cardiac rehabilitation (either exercise only or a more comprehensive lifestyle intervention including physical activity) showed a 20% reduction in all-cause mortality (hazard ratio [HR] 0.80, 95% confidence interval [CI] 0.68–0.93) and a 26% reduction in cardiac mortality (HR 0.74, 95% CI 0.61–0.96). There were no significant differences in disease outcomes between exercise only and comprehensive rehabilitation, but this comparison may be confounded by those taking exercise changing other aspects of their lifestyle.

Body Weight and Abdominal Fat

As body weight (defined as body mass index [BMI]) increases, so does the risk of CVD, but the distribution of fat, particularly visceral fat, is also an important factor. Overweight and abdominal obesity, usually measured by waist circumference in clinical practice, are associated with other risk factors including elevated BP, high LDL cholesterol, low HDL cholesterol, raised triglycerides, insulin resistance, and impaired glucose regulation, including diabetes. The clustering of risk factors, usually found in centrally obese individuals, is commonly referred to as the metabolic syndrome (see Chapter 2, page 20).

Weight reduction interventions include dietary modification, increased physical activity, and some drug treatments, all of which are effective over the short term, especially when used together. Caloric intake can be most efficiently reduced by reducing the consumption of high-energy foods, especially saturated fats, refined carbohydrates, and some alcoholic drinks, while those who are obese should restrict caloric intake as well. Fat intake should be less than 30% of total energy intake. Foods with a high fat content should be replaced with vegetables, fruit, and cereal products. A sustained weight loss of around 0.5 kg per week is a realistic objective until target weight is achieved. However, most people begin to gain weight a few months after their initial treatment. Therefore, successful weight reduction requires sustained personal and family motivation and may require long-term professional support.

Approved anti-obesity medications include inhibitors of intestinal fat absorption and those drugs that act on the central nervous system to suppress appetite, reduce food intake, increase satiety or increase thermogenesis. Obesity guidelines currently recommend that drug therapy be considered in obese people (BMI >30 kg/m^2) or in individuals with a BMI of 27–30 kg/m^2 with one or more obesity-related disorder. Clinical trials of such medications have been of short duration and the impact of these drugs on CVD and total mortality has not been assessed. Weight re-gain is common when all these drug therapies are stopped.

- In one meta-analysis, orlistat, an inhibitor of fat absorption, reduced weight by 2.7 kg (95% CI 2.3–3.1 kg) compared to placebo.
- In a 4-year trial, intensive lifestyle change supplemented with orlistat reduced the progression to diabetes by 39% compared to placebo. Gastrointestinal side effects were the most common side effect.
- In a meta-analysis, sibutramine, a centrally acting drug, reduced weight by 4.3 kg (95% CI 3.6–4.9) compared to placebo, but was associated with increases in pulse rate and BP.
- In a separate meta-analysis of sibutramine on BP, the overall effect on change in SBP was +0.16 mmHg (95% CI 0.08–0.24) and +0.26 mmHg (95% CI 0.18–0.33) for DBP.

Antihypertensive Agents

In the mid-1990s there were still several unresolved issues in the treatment of hypertension, despite the availability of results from numerous major morbidity/mortality trials to guide practice. These included:

- whether treatment with newer drugs such as calcium-channel blockers (CCBs), α-blockers, and angiotensin-converting enzyme (ACE) inhibitors resulted in greater protection against CHD events compared with the older diuretics or β-blockers;
- whether other concomitant medications would provide further benefits;
- the appropriate threshold for initiation of antihypertensive therapy and target BP levels;
- whether specific combinations of antihypertensive agents would confer benefits over other combinations; and
- the correct approach to the treatment of specific patient subgroups.

Are the Newer Agents Superior?

Following the compilation of placebo-controlled trials, the results of which were reported in (199)3 (see Fig. 3.1), a series of trials was carried

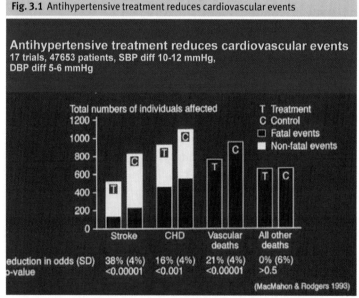

Fig. 3.1 Antihypertensive treatment reduces cardiovascular events

17 trials, 47,653 patients, systolic blood pressure difference 10–12 mmHg, diastolic blood pressure difference 5–6 mmHg. CHD, coronary heart disease; SD, standard deviation.
Reproduced with permission from MacMahon S et al. *J Vasc Med Biol* 1993; 4:265–271.

out to compare the benefits of more contemporary drugs over standard therapy. In 2000, the Blood Pressure-Lowering Treatment Trialists (BPLTT) collaboration published a meta-analysis of these trials, which included data from approximately 75,000 patients. It is important to emphasize that all eligible trials had to conform to pre-specified criteria and the collaborators agreed to a program of prospectively designed overviews.

The main conclusion from this important analysis was that overall CV events were not differentially influenced by different treatment regimens based on older or newer drugs. However, there were still too few patients to allow definitive conclusions to be drawn about the lack of benefits of any particular treatment regimen. In addition, no analyses had been undertaken on particular patient subgroups.

However, certain trends were noted; for example, there appeared to be fewer stroke events and more CHD events with CCB regimens than the more established drugs (see Fig. 3.2). There were no significant differences observed between regimens based on ACE inhibitors compared with those based on diuretics or β-blockers, except for the expected trend in favor of ACE inhibitors in treating heart failure.

The findings from the most recent meta-analyses from the BPLTT collaboration in 2003 are consistent with those from 2000, showing that the main source of benefit from BP-lowering drugs is reduced BP itself (i.e., there was little evidence of any additional class-specific benefits over and above the BP-lowering effect). In summary, the conclusions of the 2003 analyses were as follows:

Fig. 3.2 First blood pressure-lowering treatment trials (BPLTT) collaboration meta-analysis

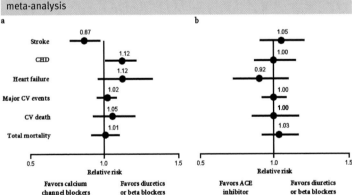

(a) Calcium-channel blockers versus diuretics/β-blockers. (b) Angiotensin-converting enzyme (ACE) inhibitors versus diuretics/β-blockers. CHD, coronary heart disease; CV, cardiovascular. Adapted from Neal B et al. *Lancet* 2000; 356:1955–1964.

- similar net effects on total CV events of ACE inhibitors, CCBs, and diuretics/β-blockers;
- angiotensin receptor blockers (ARBs) are also effective in reducing total CV events;
- ACE inhibitors and diuretics/ β-blockers are more effective than CCBs in preventing heart failure;
- CCBs may be more effective for stroke prevention;
- more intensive BP lowering produces large reductions in stroke and total CV events;
- the size of BP difference between randomized groups is closely associated with reduction in risk (except for heart failure); and
- the extent of BP reduction appears to be a more important determinant of outcome than drug choice.

Recently, three further issues have arisen suggesting differential benefits amongst the major antihypertensive agents:

1. *Stroke protection* – Two recent meta-analyses have demonstrated that β-blockers appear to be less effective than other antihypertensive agents at preventing strokes. These data, along with other considerations, have precipitated changes in British guidelines such that β-blockers are now relegated to fourth-line agents except where compelling indications apply (see discussion under *Combining antihypertensive agents*, page 34 and accompanying Fig. 3.9).
2. *Diabetegenicity* – One of the other major issues that precipitated the most recent changes in BHS hypertension guidance was the differential effects of the major drug classes on the development of new-onset diabetes (NOD). Recent compilations of trial data have been consistent in showing that both diuretics and β-blockers generate an increased risk of NOD compared with other agents. Meanwhile, evidence has gradually accumulated to suggest that ACE inhibitors and ARBs may protect against the development of NOD whilst CCBs appear to be neutral from this viewpoint. Evidence from trials are as yet too few and of too short duration to show that drug-induced NOD is associated with increased risk of CVD. However, pending such data, it seems clear that NOD should be avoided and the differential effects of the antihypertensive drug classes on NOD should be considered.
3. *Benefits beyond BP* – This issue has been contentious for several years. It is clear from the extensive meta-analyses produced by the BPLTT

collaboration that there is a strong correlation between CV outcomes and degree of BP reduction. However, inconsistencies do exist and, given the multifactorial etiology of different CV events and the differential impact of various antihypertensive agents on established CV risk factors (other than BP) and on duration of BP-lowering action, it seems unlikely that all antihypertensives would exert the same CV benefits for the same degree of clinic BP reduction.

These conclusions were supported by analyses of the Anglo-Scandinavian Cardiac Outcomes trial–Blood Pressure-Lowering Arm (ASCOT-BPLA) trial, in which a newer antihypertensive regimen (amlodipine +/– perindopril) was superior to an older regimen (atenolol +/– thiazide) in terms of preventing death, total coronary events, strokes, and total CV events and procedures (see discussion under *Combining antihypertensive agents*, page 3(3) and accompanying Fig. 3.13). Although these differences did occur in the face of a small superior BP-lowering effect of the newer regimen, analyses suggested that the different CV event rates were unlikely to be due to better BP control alone.

The findings of a recent meta-analysis also fully supports the ASCOT-BPLA results in this regard by showing that ACE inhibitors appear to provide additional prevention of CHD events over and above BP lowering, and that CCBs provide prevention of stroke events over and above BP lowering (see Fig. 3.3).

Administration of Antihypertensive Agents: Practical Issues

Assuming a suitable period of assessment (between 3 weeks and 6 months—the duration being inversely related to the severity of the BP readings) and that non-pharmacological measures have been attempted and found to be insufficient, the national and international management guidelines agree about the following general issues relating to drug therapy:

- either SBP or DBP criteria for treatment should be considered;
- drug therapy should be considered at least up to the age of 80 years and one recently completed trail, HYVET, has confirmed the benefits of treatment above his age;
- early and/or urgent treatment of severe and/or malignant hypertension;
- thresholds for drug intervention should be lower for those with established target organ damage (e.g., CVD, LVH, renal disease) or diabetes than among those without such risk factors; and
- BP-lowering regimens should attempt to reach specified targets.

Fig. 3.3 ACE inhibitors and CCBs further reduce the risk of CHD and stroke

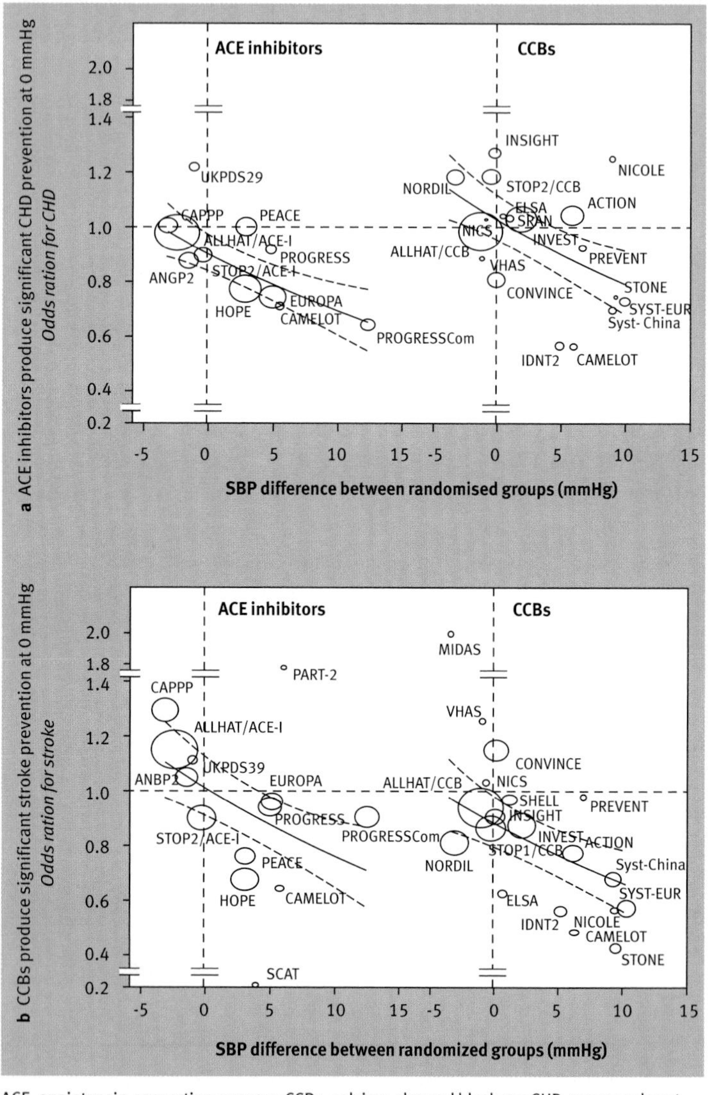

ACE, angiotensin-converting enzyme; CCBs, calcium-channel blockers; CHD, coronary heart disease; SBP, systolic blood pressure. Circles represent individual trials and have a diameter proportional to the inverse of the variance of the odds ratios in individual trials. Reproduced with permission from Verdecchia P et al. *Hypertension* 2005; 46:386–392.

When to Treat

It is clear from trial evidence that important clinical benefits accrue from treating SBP ⩾160 mmHg or DBP ⩾100 mmHg. Evidence for the benefits of treating lowering levels of BP at least among low risk people is less clear. Nevertheless, on the basis of prospective data, current guidelines recommend that thresholds for intervention are lowered for patients with target organ damage, established vascular disease, diabetes, or those above certain estimated levels of coronary or CV risk. Consequently, as described in Chapter 2, assessment charts have been developed to facilitate this approach of identifying risk levels among hypertensive patients.

Current British guidelines are among the most conservative in the world in recommending antihypertensive treatment to all those with an SBP ⩾160 mmHg or DBP ⩾100 mmHg and among those with an SBP ⩾140–159 mmHg or DBP ⩾90–99 mmHg who have either target organ damage (e.g., LVH), established vascular disease, or an estimated 10-year CVD risk of ⩾20% (see Fig. 3.4). These recommendations are shown together with other international guidelines in Table 3.2.

Advantages, Disadvantages, and Common Side Effects of the Major Drug Classes

The advantages, disadvantages, and common side effects of the six main drug classes are shown in Table 3.3, and some examples of patient profiling, as suggested in the most recent BHS and WHO–ISH guidelines, are shown in Table 3.4.

Combining Antihypertensive Agents

Results from almost all the major trials, including the Hypertension Optimal Treatment (HOT) trial and the UK Prospective Diabetes Study (UKPDS), show that the majority of patients with hypertension require at least two BP-lowering agents if the current recommended targets are to be reached (see Fig. 3.5).

Although most antihypertensive drug trials have involved the use of BP-lowering regimens with two or more agents, the choice of a second or third agent has usually been unstructured and therefore cannot provide recommendations for optimal drug combinations. Doctors have been recommended to select drugs with complementary rather than overlapping mechanisms of action (see Fig. 3.6). More recently, in 2003 ESH–ESC guidelines produced an updated version of these earlier suggestions (see Fig. 3.7).

It is worth highlighting that these latest European guidelines contradict earlier recommendations in that CCBs and diuretics are considered to be a logical combination, despite sharing some similarities in their mechanism

Fig. 3.4 Risk targets and thresholds for blood pressure for asymptomic people without CVD

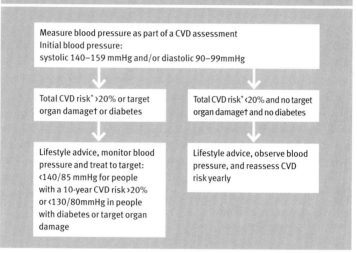

Measure blood pressure as part of a CVD assessment
Initial blood pressure:
systolic 140–159 mmHg and/or diastolic 90–99mmHg

Total CVD risk*>20% or target organ damage† or diabetes

Total CVD risk*<20% and no target organ damage† and no diabetes

Lifestyle advice, monitor blood pressure and treat to target: <140/85 mmHg for people with a 10-year CVD risk >20% or <130/80mmHg in people with diabetes or target organ damage

Lifestyle advice, observe blood pressure, and reassess CVD risk yearly

*Assessed with cardiovascular (CVD) risk chart. †Heart failure, established coronary heart disease, stroke, transient ischemic attack, peripheral arterial disease, abnormal renal function (elevated serum creatinine or proteinuria/microalbuminuria), hypertensive or diabetic retinopathy, left ventricular hypertrophy on ECG or echocardiography. Reproduced with permission from the JBS 2 guidelines. *Heart* 2005; 91(Suppl 5):1–52.

Table 3.2 ESH-ESC Guidelines 2007

Other risk factors OD or disease	Blood pressure (mmHg)				
	Normal SBP 120–129 or DBP 80–84	High normal SBP 130–139 or DBP 85–89	Grade 1 HT SBP 140–159 or DBP 90–99	Grade 2 HT SBP 160–179 or DBP 100–109	Grade 3 HT SBP≥180 or DBP≥110
No other risk factors	No BP intervention	No BP intervention	Lifestyle changes for several months then drug treatment if BP uncontrolled	Lifestyle changes for several weeks then drug treatment if BP uncontrolled	Lifestyle changes + Immediate drug treatment
1–2 risk factors	Lifestyle changes	Lifestyle changes	Lifestyle changes for several weeks then drug treatment if BP uncontrolled	Lifestyle changes for several weeks then drug treatment if BP uncontrolled	Lifestyle changes + Immediate drug treatment
≥3 risk factors, MS or OD	Lifestyle changes	Lifestyle changes and consider drug treatment	Lifestyle changes + Drug treatment	Lifestyle changes + Drug treatment	Lifestyle changes + Immediate drug treatment
Diabetes	Lifestyle changes	Lifestyle changes + Drug treatment			
Established CV or renal disease	Lifestyle changes + Immediate drug treatment	Lifestyle changes + Immediate drug treatment	Lifestyle changes + Immediate drug treatment	Lifestyle changes + Immediate drug treatment	Lifestyle changes + Immediate drug treatment

Initiation of antihypertensive treatment.

of action and having been shown not to produce optimal BP lowering in earlier studies. However, this combination is in common use, at least in the UK (see Table 3.5). A further change is the suggestion that α-blockers should

Table 3.3 Advantages, disadvantages, and side effects of drug treatments

Treatment	Advantages	Disadvantages	Side-effects
Diuretics	Low cost Effective in the elderly	↓ K⁺ leading to arrhythmias ? glucose ↑ cholesterol and triglyerides ↑ uric acid	Impotence Urinary frequency Gout
Beta-Blockers	Good for angina, Good for anxiety, Good for post-MI	↑ triglycerides ↓ HDL cholesterol ↓ cardiac output/exercise tolerance Contraindicated in asthma; caution in CCF and PVD ? Reduced stroke protection	Lethargy Raynaud's phenomenon Sleep disturbance Depression Impotence
ACE inhibitors	LVH regression ↓ Na⁺ retention Lipid neutral Renal protection in diabetes	Contraindicated in renal artery stenosis and women of child-bearing age	Cough Hypotension (with diuretic)
All antagonists	Well tolerated (no ACE cough)	As for ACE inhibitors	Hypotension (with diuretic)
CCBs	Lipid neutral Weak diuretic effect Anti-anginal effect	Negative inotropic effect of verapamil and diltiazem Short-acting drugs contraindicated in CHD	Flushing Headaches Oedema
Alpha-blockers	Improvement in lipid profile and insulin resistance improved sexual potency Improved prostatism	Caution in heart failure	Palpitations Postural hypotension (with short-acting agents)

ACE, angiotensin-converting enzyme; CCBs, calcium-channel blockers; CCF, congestive cardiac failure; DHP, dihydropyridine; HDL, high-density lipoprotein; LVH, left ventricular hypertrophy; MI, myocardial infarction; PVD, peripheral vascular disease.

not be used in combination with any other agent except β-blockers and ACE inhibitors. Although this change may have emerged from the findings of ALLHAT (Antihypertensive and Lipid-Lowering Treatment to Prevent Heart Attack Trial), the study's design does not allow for conclusions on drug combinations and, therefore, α-blockers should probably be regarded as complementary with all other drug classes.

The BHS has, until recently, proposed the ABCD algorithm as a way to best combine antihypertensive agents to achieve optimal BP control

Table 3.4 Compelling and possible indications, contraindications, and cautions for the major classes of antihypertensive drugs

Class of drug	Compelling indications	Possible indications	Caution	Compelling contraindications
α-Blockers	Benign prostatic hypertrophy		Postural hypotension, heart failure*	Urinary incontinence
ACE inhibitors	Heart failure, LV dysfunction, post MI or established CHD, type I diabetic nephropathy, secondary stroke prevention¶	Chronic renal disease,† type II diabetic nephropathy, proteinuric renal disease	Renal impairment‡ PVD‡	Pregnancy, renovascular disease§
ARBs	ACE inhibitor intolerance, type II diabetic nephropathy, hypertension with LVH, heart failure in ACE-intolerant patients, post MI	LV dysfunction post MI, intolerance of other antihypertensive drugs, proteinuric renal disease, chronic renal disease, heart failure†	Renal impairment† PVD‡	Pregnancy, renovascular disease§
β-Blockers	MI, angina	Heart failure#	Heart failure#, PVD, diabetes (except with CHD)	Asthma/COPD, heart block
CCBs (DHP)	Elderly, ISH	Elderly, angina	–	–
CCBs (rate limiting)	Angina	MI	Combination with β-blockade	Heart block, heart failure
Thiazide/ thiazide-like diuretics	Elderly, ISH, heart failure, secondary stroke prevention			Gout**

CCB, calcium-channel blocker; CHD, coronary heart disease; COPD, chronic obstructive pulmonary disease; DHP, dihydropyridine; ISH, isolate systolic hypertension; LV, left ventricular; LVH, left ventricular hypertrophy; MI, myocardial infarction. *Heart failure when used as monotherapy. †Angiotensin-coverting enzyme (ACE) inhibitors or angiotensin II receptor blockers (ARBs) may be beneficial in chronic renal failure but should only be used with caution, close supervision, and specialist advice when there is established and significant renal impairment. ‡Caution with ACE inhibitors and ARBs in peripheral vascular disease (PVD) because of association with renovascular disease (RVD). §ACE inhibitors and ARBs are sometimes used in patients with RVD under specialist supervision. ¶In combination with a thiazide/thiazide-like diuretic. #-blockers are increasingly used to treat stable heart failure; however, -blockers may worsen heart failure. **Thiazide/thiazide-like diuretics may sometimes be necessary to control blood pressure in people with a history of gout, ideally used in combination with allopurinol. Reproduced with permission from the JBS 2 guidelines. *Heart* 2005; 91(Suppl 5):1–52.

Fig. 3.5 Combination therapy is needed to achieve target blood pressure (HOT study)

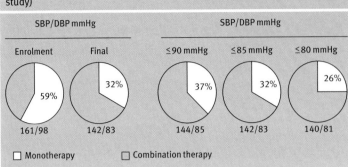

DBP, diastolic blood pressure; HOT, Hypertension Optimal Treatment; SBP, systolic blood pressure. Adapted from Hansson L et al. *Lancet* 1998; 351:1755–1762.

Fig. 3.6 Combination therapy needed to achieve target blood pressure

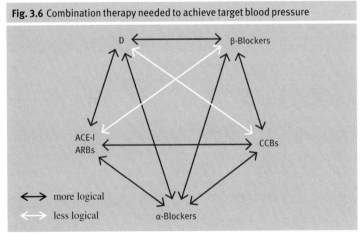

ACE-I, angiotensin-converting enzyme inhibitor; ARBs, angiotensin receptor blockers; CCBs, calcium-channel blockers; D, diuretic. Reproduced with permission from Cappuccio FP et al. *J Hum Hypertens* 1991; 5(Suppl 2):9–15.

(see Fig. 3.8). This approach is based on the theory that hypertension can be broadly classified as "high renin," which is best treated by those drug classes that inhibit the renin-angiotensin system (i.e., ACE inhibitors/ARBs or β-blockers), or "low renin," which should be treated by drug classes that do not inhibit the system (i.e., CCBs or diuretics).

Caucasians under 55 years of age tend to have higher renin status than black or older people, providing the rationale for step 1. The rationale for

Fig. 3.7 Possible two-drug combination therapy as suggested by ESH–ESC

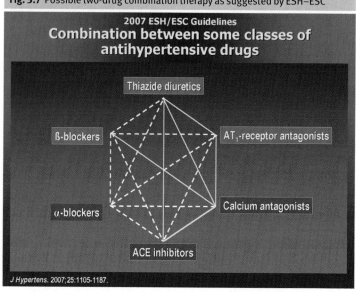

ACE-I, angiotensin-converting enzyme inhibitor inhibitors; ARBs, angiotensin
receptor blockers; CCBs, calcium-channel blockers; ESH–ESC, European Society of
Hypertension–European Society of Cardiology. Reproduced from ESH–ESC guidelines.
J Hypertens 2003; 21:1011–1053.

Table 3.5 Combinations of antihypertensive therapy use in the UK

Drugs	1994 (%)	1998 (%)	2003 (%)
Diuretic + β-blocker	41 ± 2.5	21 ± 1.93	21 ± 1.7
Diuretic + CCB	19 ± 2.0	21 ± 1.93	16 ± 1.6
Diuretic + ACE inhibitor	15 ± 1.8	27 ± 2.1	24 ± 1.8
Other	25 ± 2.2	31 ± 2.2	39 ± 2.1

ACE, angiotensin-converting enzyme; CCB, calcium-channel blocker.
Adapted from Primatesta P et al. *Hypertension* 2001; 38:827–832.

steps 2, 3, and 4 is based on the logical grounds of avoiding combinations
of agents that have overlapping mechanisms of action. This algorithm has
the added advantage of providing advice on how best to control more severe
levels of raised BP. For those patients with apparently resistant hypertension
despite taking several conventional agents, the use of aldosterone antagonists
(e.g., spironolactone 25 mg od) appears to provide dramatic BP-lowering
effects.

Fig. 3.8 The BHS recommentations for combining blood pressure-lowering drugs

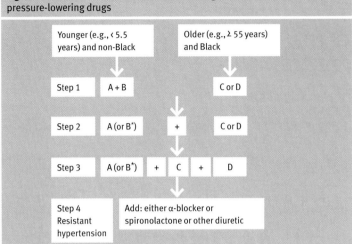

*Combination therapy involving B and D may induce more new-onset diabetes compared with other combination therapies. A, angiotensin-converting enzyme inhibitor or angiotensin receptor blocker; B, β-blocker; C, calcium-channel blocker; D, thiazide/ thiazide-type diuretic. Adapted from Brown MJ et al. *J Hum Hypertens* 2003; 17:81–86.

More recently, in light of the ASCOT trail and recent reviews of the efficacy of β-blockers in terms of stroke prevention, the BHS has, in collaboration with the National Institute for Health and Clinical Excellence (NICE), modified their ABCD algorithm as shown in Fig. 3.9.

Recent guidelines now recommend the use of fixed low-dose combinations of drugs. Although historically this has been considered poor clinical practice, it now seems a logical approach, which should enhance compliance and BP lowering. With this in mind, the JNC 7 and the latest European guidelines formally recommend combination therapy as first-line treatment (see Fig. 3.10 and 3.11).

Despite the need to use two drugs or more for BP control in most patients, the ASCOT trial is the only trial reporting before 2008 which was specifically designed to compare the effects of two totally different combinations of anti-hypertensive treatment (see Fig. 3.12).

This trial showed that the use of an antihypertensive regimen based on the CCB amlodipine, and adding the ACE inhibitor perindopril as required to reach BP targets (<140/90 mmHg for non-diabetics and <130/80 for diabetics), was superior to a regimen based on the β-blocker atenolol and adding the thiazide bendroflumethiazide as required, in terms of all major

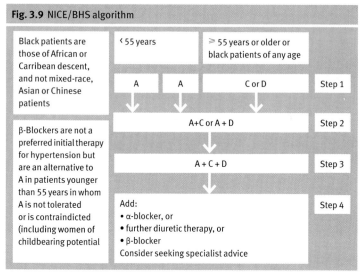

Fig. 3.9 NICE/BHS algorithm

A, angiotensin-converting enzyme inhibitor or angiotensin receptor blocker; B, C, calcium-channel blocker; D, thiazide/thiazide-type diuretic. NICE 2006 guidelines Hypertension: Managers of hypertension adults i primary care

CV events and all-cause mortality. The extent to which the result was driven by marginally different BP lowering in the two treatment groups remains controversial. However, the authors suggest that the BP difference in favour of amoldipine of perindopril (2.7/1.9 mmHg) was probably insufficient to explain the considerable differences in CV events shown in Fig. 3.13. More recently the ACOMPLISH trail has shown for almost identical BF lowing than an A+C combination was superior to an A+D combination in terms of preventing major CV events.

Lipid-Lowering Agents

Before the uptake of statins, a meta-analysis of lipid-lowering trials showed that a 10% reduction in plasma total cholesterol, whether by diet or drugs and whether in primary or secondary prevention, was associated with over a 20% reduction in CHD incidence after 5 years.

More recently, an extensive body of evidence has accrued from trials of statin use for the prevention of all CV events. These data showing large important benefits in terms of CVD prevention apply in the context of primary and secondary prevention for men, women, those with and without

Fig. 3.10 Algorithm for treatment of hypertension in JNC 7

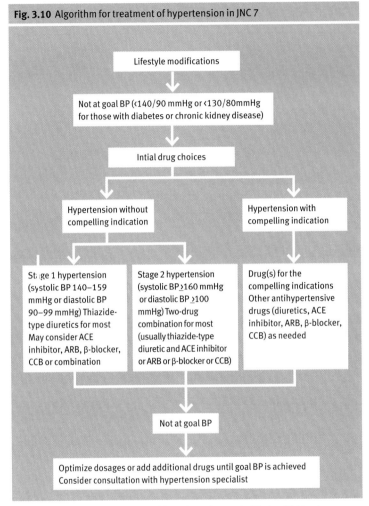

ACE, angiotensin-converting enzyme; ARB, angiotensin receptor blocker; BP, blood pressure; CCB, calcium-channel blocker. Reproduced with permission from Chobanian AV et al. *Hypertension* 2003; 42:1206–1252.

diabetes or hypertension, young or old, and these benefits are irrespective of baseline lipid levels (see Fig. 3.14).

The most recent comprehensive meta-analyses of these data show that all CV events are reduced in association with statin use, as is all-cause mortality (see Fig. 3.15).

Fig. 3.11 ESH–ESC algorithm for treatment of hypertension

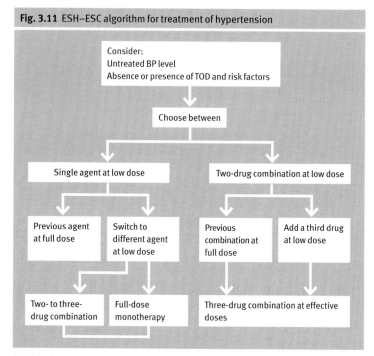

ABP, blood pressure; TOD, target organ damage. Reproduced with permission from ESH–ESC guidelines. *J Hypertens* 2003; 21:1011–1053.

Fig. 3.12 ASCOT study design

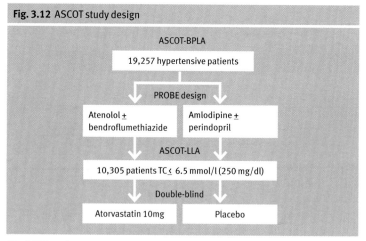

LLA, lipid-lowering arm; TC, total cholesterol. Adapted from Sever PS et al. ASCOT-BPLA: The Anglo-Scandinavian Cardiac Outcomes Trial: Blood Pressure-Lowering Arm. Poulter NR et al. Lancet 2005: 336:907–913.

Fig. 3.13 Effect of treatment on all ASCOT-BPLA endpoints

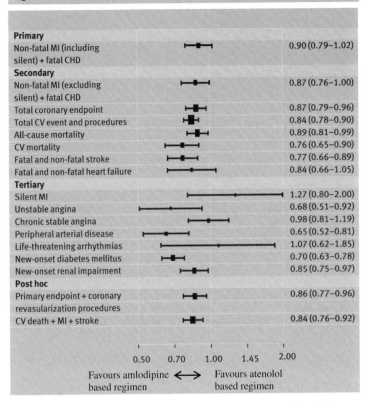

Primary		
Non-fatal MI (including silent) + fatal CHD		0.90 (0.79–1.02)
Secondary		
Non-fatal MI (excluding silent) + fatal CHD		0.87 (0.76–1.00)
Total coronary endpoint		0.87 (0.79–0.96)
Total CV event and procedures		0.84 (0.78–0.90)
All-cause mortality		0.89 (0.81–0.99)
CV mortality		0.76 (0.65–0.90)
Fatal and non-fatal stroke		0.77 (0.66–0.89)
Fatal and non-fatal heart failure		0.84 (0.66–1.05)
Tertiary		
Silent MI		1.27 (0.80–2.00)
Unstable angina		0.68 (0.51–0.92)
Chronic stable angina		0.98 (0.81–1.19)
Peripheral arterial disease		0.65 (0.52–0.81)
Life-threatening arrhythmias		1.07 (0.62–1.85)
New-onset diabetes mellitus		0.70 (0.63–0.78)
New-onset renal impairment		0.85 (0.75–0.97)
Post hoc		
Primary endpoint + coronary revasularization procedures		0.86 (0.77–0.96)
CV death + MI + stroke		0.84 (0.76–0.92)

0.50   0.70   1.00   1.45   2.00

Favours amlodipine ←→ Favours atenolol
based regimen   based regimen

CHD, coronary heart disease; CI, confidence interval; CV, cardiovascular; HR, hazard ratio; MI, myocardial infarction. Reproduced with permission from Dahlof B et al. *Lancet* 2005; 366:895–906.

The only exceptional endpoint was hemorrhagic stroke, for which no significant benefit or harm was apparent. Interestingly, since this meta-analysis, the first trial of statin use for the secondary prevention of stroke (SPARCL) has reported significant benefits on all stroke events, although, once again, no significant adverse impact on hemorrhagic stroke was apparent. Reassuringly from the meta-analysis, statin use was not associated with any increase of any type of death, nor of any cancers. The criteria for thresholds for intervention with statins varies from the type of patient as described below.

Fig. 3.14 Absolute risk reduction with changes in LDL

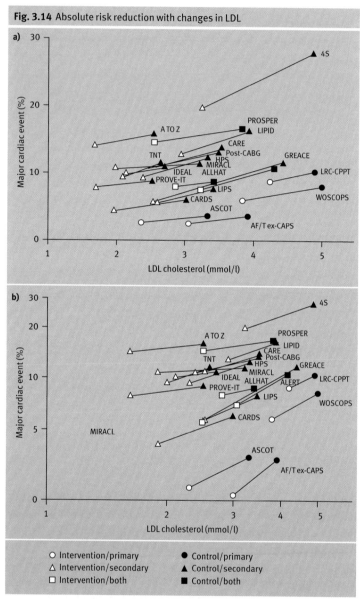

(a) Absolute reduction in low-density lipoprotein (LDL) cholesterol (mmol/l) and absolute reduction in risk of major cardiac event. (b) Both axes are on a log scale showing relative reduction in LDL cholesterol (mmol/l) and relative reduction in risk of major cardiac event. Reproduced with permission from JBS 2 guidelines. *Heart* 2005; 91:(Suppl 5)1–52.

Fig. 3.15 Proportional effects on major CVD events per 1 mmol/L LDL reduction

Endpoint	Events (%)			RR (CI)
	Treatment (45,054)	**Control (45,002)**		
Non-fatal MI	2001 (4.4%)	2769 (6.2%)		0.74 (0.70–0.79)
CHD death	1548 (3.4%)	1960 (4.4%)		0.81 (0.75–0.87)
Any major coronary event	3337 (7.4%)	4420 (9.8%)		0.77 (0.74–0.80)
CABG	713 (1.6%)	1006 (2.2%)		0.75 (0.69–0.82)
PTCA	510 (1.1%)	658 (1.5%)		0.79 (0.69–0.90)
Unspecified	1397 (3.1%)	1770 (3.9%)		0.76 (0.69–0.84)
Any coronary revascularization	2620 (5.8%)	3434 (7.6%)		0.76 (0.73–0.80)
Hemorrhagic stroke	105 (0.2%)	99 (0.2%)		1.05 (0.78–1.41)
Presumed ischemic stroke	1235 (2.8%)	1518 (3.4%)		0.81 (0.74–0.89)
Any stroke	1340 (3.0%)	1617 (3.7%)		0.83 (0.78–0.88)
Any major vascular event	6354 (14.1%)	7994 (17.8%)		0.79 (0.77–0.81)

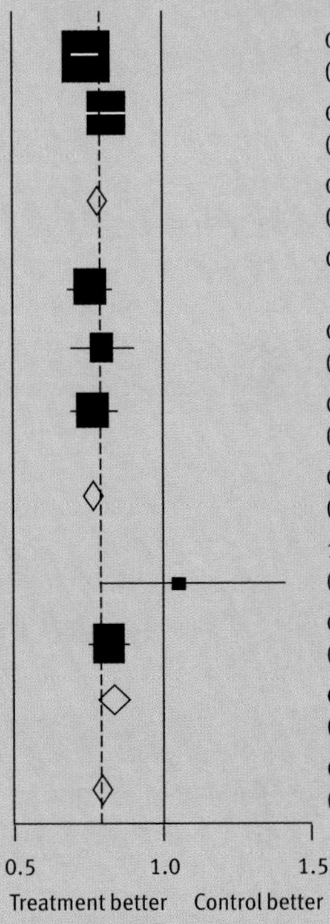

0.5   1.0   1.5

Treatment better   Control better

Effect *p*<0.0001

CABG, coronary artery bypass graft; CHD, coronary heart disease; CV, cardiovascular; MI, myocardial infarction; PTCA, percutaneous transluminal coronary angioplasty. *Diamonds* equal totals and subtotals (95% confidence interval [CI]). *Squares* equal individual categories (*horizontal lines* are 99% CI). Area of square proportional to amount of statistical information in that category. *Broken vertical line* indicates overall rate ratio (RR) for any type of major vascular event. Reproduced with permission from Cholesterol Treatment Trialists" collaborators. *Lancet* 2005; 366:1267–1278.

When to Start Therapy?

People with Coronary and Other Atherosclerotic Diseases

Although the traditional approach has been to start with dietary advice and then consider lipid-lowering therapy some months after the acute event, there have been three clinical trials assessing the impact of starting statin treatment early. However, only one of these—the MIRACL (Myocardial Ischemia Reduction with Aggressive Cholesterol Lowering) trial—is a placebo-controlled trial to assess the short-term impact of immediate treatment. The evidence from these three trials supports the view that early in-hospital statin treatment is of benefit in reducing the risk of further CV events in the short term.

Therefore, the current recommendation is that all people with acute atherosclerotic (coronary, cerebral, and peripheral) disease, but not cerebral hemorrhage, should be prescribed a statin in hospital regardless of the initial cholesterol value. The rationale for this policy is as follows:

- The three trials of early initiation of statin treatment show some evidence of early CV benefit.
- The vast majority of such people will have a total cholesterol ⩾4.0 mmol/l (LDL cholesterol ⩾2.0 mmol/l) and, therefore, most will require a statin to achieve and maintain lipid targets.
- Measurement of lipids in the acute phase of the disease will usually underestimate the pre-disease values, and therefore are not usually an accurate guide to therapy at this point. So a total cholesterol below the target of 4.0 mmol/l in the acute situation is not a reason to delay treatment with a statin.
- It emphasizes to the person with the disease the importance of lipid lowering, by both lifestyle and drug intervention, for their future CV health.
- Starting treatment in hospital is more likely to result in the same treatment being continued in general practice.

There will be clinical exceptions to this policy—for example, a person with stroke-related dementia and acute atherosclerotic disease may not be suitable for statin treatment. Assessment for secondary causes of dyslipidemia should take place at the same time. Fasting lipids should be measured about 8–12 weeks after the acute event, and drug therapy appropriately modified to ensure lipid targets are achieved.

People with Diabetes Mellitus

People with diabetes mellitus (without CVD) should have their fasting lipids measured, and be given diet and lifestyle advice. If total cholesterol remains ≥3.5 mmol/l then lifestyle advice should be reinforced and a statin is indicated for all those aged ≥40 with either type 1 or 2 diabetes or people aged 18–39 with either type 1 or 2 diabetes and who have at least one of the following:

- retinopathy (pre-proliferative, proliferative, maculopathy);
- nephropathy, including persistent microalbuminuria;
- poor glycemic control (HbA1c >9%);
- elevated BP requiring antihypertensive therapy;
- raised total blood cholesterol (≥6.0 mmol/l);
- features of metabolic syndrome (central obesity and fasting triglyceride >1.7 mmol/l [non-fasting >2.0 mmol/l] and/or HDL cholesterol >1.0 mmol/l in men or >1.2 mmol/l in women); or
- family history of premature CVD in a first-degree relative.

Although the most common form of dyslipidemia in diabetes is low HDL cholesterol and elevated triglycerides, the roles of fibrates and the nicotinic acid group are still unclear and a statin is the drug class of first choice. However, low HDL cholesterol and elevated triglycerides may also require treatment once the total and LDL cholesterol targets are achieved.

People at high total CVD risk

For asymptomatic people who are at high total risk of developing CVD (≥20% over 10 years), a guide for the management of lipids is provided in Fig. 3.16.

Familial Dyslipidemias

Familial hypercholesterolemia (FH) is an autosomal-dominant disorder with an estimated prevalence of 1 in 500 of the adult population. The criteria for the diagnosis of FH are given via PRODIGY (see www.prodigy.nhs.uk). In people with FH, angina or acute coronary syndromes (non-fatal and fatal) typically occur in men aged between 30 and 50 years and in women between 50 and 70 years and have a CHD mortality rate at least 10 times greater than the general population. Early identification of people with FH should result in appropriate professional lifestyle intervention, treatment with a statin and, where necessary, other lipid-lowering therapies. All first-degree relatives of people with premature CHD (men <55 years and women <65 years) should be screened for lipids. Guidelines for children with FH are given in the joint

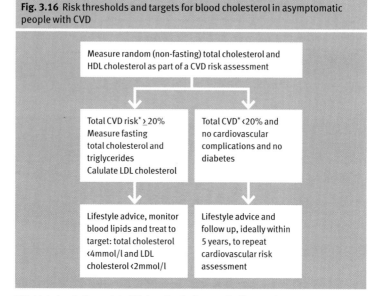

Fig. 3.16 Risk thresholds and targets for blood cholesterol in asymptomatic people with CVD

Measure random (non-fasting) total cholesterol and HDL cholesterol as part of a CVD risk assessment

Total CVD risk* ≥ 20%
Measure fasting total cholesterol and triglycerides
Calulate LDL cholesterol

Total CVD* ‹20% and no cardiovascular complications and no diabetes

Lifestyle advice, monitor blood lipids and treat to target: total cholesterol ‹4mmol/l and LDL cholesterol ‹2mmol/l

Lifestyle advice and follow up, ideally within 5 years, to repeat cardiovascular risk assessment

HDL, high-density lipoprotein; LDL, low-density lipoprotein. *Assessed with cardiovascular disease (CVD) risk chart. Reproduced from the JBS 2 guidelines. *Heart* 2005; 91(Suppl 5): 1–52.

publication of the former British Hyperlipidaemia Association and the British Paediatric Association on Paediatric Hyperlipidaemia, but people with FH and their families should be looked after by lipid specialists.

Familial combined hyperlipidemia (FCH) is a heterogeneous group of lipid disorders with a variable inheritance pattern and a prevalence of at least 1 in 300 of the adult population. FCH is characterized by raised cholesterol and/or triglycerides as well as premature CHD in family members.

Selection of Drug Therapies

The compelling and possible indications, contraindications, and cautions for the major lipid-modifying drugs are shown in Table 3.6. Lipids and lipoproteins may be influenced by other drugs such as insulin, metformin, thiazolidinediones, orlistat, and sibutramine.

Statins

The HMG-CoA reductase inhibitor (statin) class is the most potent of the lipid-lowering drug classes for lowering both total and LDL cholesterol. Statins are administered once daily with few side effects and have a good

Table 3.6 Compelling and possible indications, contraindications, and cautions for the major classes of lipid-lowering drugs

Class of drug	Compelling indications	Possible indications	Caution	Compelling contraindications
Anion exchange resins	None (because of poor gastrointestinal tolerability)	Inadequate LDL-C control on statin and ezetimibe (e.g., familial hypercholesterolemia) Cholestasis with itching	Gastrointestinal upset Exacerbation of hypertriglyceridemia Interaction with other drugs Reduction in fat soluble vitamin absorption (not normally clinically significant)	None
Cholesterol absorption inhibitors	Familial sitosterolemia	With a statin where LDL-C is not at target despite maximum licensed statin dose or maximum tolerated statin dose Statin intolerance	Liver impairment With fibrates except on specialist clinics	None
Fibrates	Type III hyperlipoproteinemia (familial dysbetalipoproteinemia, remnant lipemia)	Type 2 diabetes mellitus with raised triglycerides and low HDL-C on specialist advice Moderate–severe hypertriglyceridemia with controlled LDL-C and particularly elevated CVD risk on specialist advice	Chronic renal failure Concurrent statin therapy	Never use gemfibrozil with a statin
Fish oils: omega-3 acid ethylesters (eicosapentenoic, docosahexenoic and a-tocopherol); omega-3 marine triglycerides	Severe hypertriglyceridemia (>10 mmol/l) where there is a risk of pancreatitis	Treatment of hypertriglyceridemia	Anticoagulants Haemorrhagic disorders Aspirin-sensitive asthma Diabetes mellitus	None

Table 3.6 Compelling and possible indications, contraindictions and cautiouns for the major classes of lipid-lowering drugs

Class of drug	Compelling indications	Possible indications	Caution	Compelling contraindications
HMG-CoA reductase inhibitors (statins)	Atherosclerotic cardiovascular disease • Type 1 and 2 diabetes mellitus aged 40 years or more, or • Type 1 or 2 diabetes mellitus aged 18–39 years with specific indications (see page 47) CVD risk >20% 10 years Familial hypercholesterolemia	CVD 10–20% 10 years if: • Cholesterol/HDL ratio >6, or • LDL-C >5 mmol/l	Non-alcoholic steatohepatitis Untreated hyperthyroidism Significant chronic renal impairment (creatinine >160 μmol/l) Certain drugs and large amounts of grapefruit juice metabolized through cytochrome P450, especially 3A4 Excess alcohol intake	Gemfibrozil Significant liver disease (moderate transaminase elevation up to three times upper limit of normal may represent fatty change and not be a contraindication)
Nicotinic acid group (lipid-regulating doses)	Severe hypertriglyceridemia with prior acute pancreatitis Type V (severe hypertriglyceridemia not responsive to fibrates)	In combination with other lipid-regulating drugs to reduce both cholesterol and triglycerides Most often used in mixed hyperlipidemia	Other lipid-lowering drugs Impaired renal function Liver disease Diabetes mellitus Gout Peptic ulcer Flushing, diarrhoea as side effects	Worsening glucose tolerance Diarrhoea and/or flushing

(Continued.) CVD, cardiovascular disease; HDL-C, high-density lipoprotein cholesterol; HMG-CoA, 3-hydroxy-3-methylglutaryl coenzyme A; LDL-C, low-density lipoprotein cholesterol. Adapted from the JBS 2 guidelines. *Heart* 2005; 91(Suppl 5):1–52.

long-term safety record. Their principal effect is to lower LDL cholesterol, but they also raise HDL cholesterol and lower triglycerides to some extent. The statins are first-line drugs for reducing total and LDL cholesterol and have the most convincing trial evidence for preventing CVD events of any of the lipid-lowering drug classes.

Other Agents
Other lipid-lowering drugs will be required in some people, usually in combination with a statin if the total and LDL cholesterol targets are not achieved with a statin alone, or in place of a statin when the primary lipid abnormality is severe hypertriglyceridemia (>10 mmol/l), or when people are intolerant of statins.

Combination Statin–Fibrate Therapy
Only one large RCT with a Statin and a fibrate in combination has yet been published, with relatively disappointing results. For most people with both elevated cholesterol and triglycerides, treatment should still start with a statin. Where persistent hypertriglyceridemia is present after LDL targets are achieved, a combination of a statin with a fibrate (using fenofibrate, bezafibrate, or ciprofibrate) can be considered on specialist advice. Gemfibrozil should not be used in combination with a statin. When a statin–fibrate combination is used, monitoring of creatine kinase and alanine aminotransferase is appropriate.

Combination of Statins with Inhibitors of Cholesterol Absorption
Ezetimibe is well tolerated in combination with statins, but the long-term safety and outcome trial data with this new class of drug are at best disappointing.

Combination Treatments
There is a continuing need for more effective agents from among currently available cholesterol or BP-lowering drug classes, ideally with fewer side effects. Perhaps more importantly, newer classes of agents are being developed. To provide real advances over currently available agents, such products will need to have a long duration of action and low side-effect rates, with cholesterol or BP-lowering efficacy associated with commensurate reduction in CV events. The benefits of pharmacogenetics, whereby drugs may be targeted on the basis of genetic profiling, are considered by some to be on the horizon, although others believe it to be a rather distant horizon. Meanwhile, with the increasing need and use of polypharmacy in an ageing population, the trends are likely to move further toward the use of combination therapies. This is likely to involve not just a combination of two (or more) antihypertensive

agents and, less frequently, two or more lipid-lowering agents, but also the combination of various products that act on different CV risk factors.

The need for such products is highlighted by the typical drug requirements of a diabetic patient who has suffered an MI. The minimum drug requirements for such a patient include aspirin, a statin, one (or more) oral hypoglycemic agents, a β-blocker, an ACE inhibitor or ARB, and a fish oil preparation. This patient may also need further BP-lowering agents, a fibrate, a thiazolidinedione, and insulin injections.

The STENO-2 trial was unique in evaluating the impact of multifactorial intervention. This small trial of 160 patients with type 2 diabetes and microalbuminuria compared "usual care" with more aggressive intervention on lifestyle and with drugs for BP-, lipid-, and glucose-lowering, and with drugs targeted at microalbuminuria (ACE inhibitor or ARB) and aspirin.

After nearly 8 years of follow-up the intensive group showed highly significant benefits in terms of CVD events, stroke, amputations, microvascular events, and neuropathy. More recently, longer-term follow-up has confirmed benefits in terms of all-cause mortality.

It is obvious that compliance would be enhanced by combining some of these products into one tablet, a concept that has been highlighted recently in an article proposing the production of a "polypill," which includes several different drug types. In the context of high-risk patients (e.g., those with raised BP) a logical combination might include one or more effective BP-lowering agents, a lipid-lowering agent, and low-dose aspirin. However, the requirements of a polypill for use in a population strategy—that is to give to everyone above a certain age—are more stringent. In short, the components should have a side-effect profile that is as close to that of a placebo as possible, because the risk–benefit ratio becomes less favorable at the population level. Large reductions in each of the risk factors to be targeted are not required, but the benefits of each of the components must have been established in large RCTs.

Of currently available products, the combination of an ARB, a statin, a CCB and more contraversially a very low-dose aspirin would best suit the ideal requirements of a polypill for use in the whole population aged ≥ 50 years. However, the composition of the polypill that was recently proposed does not fit the ideal profile of such an agent because of the six agents to be combined; it includes folate (unproven to produce any CV benefits in trials as yet) and, β-blockers, ACE inhibitors and diuretics (these three drug classes are variably associated with frequent side effects including weight gain, small adverse lipid and glucose effects, wheezing in those with obstructive airways disease, cough, impotence, and urinary frequency). Furthermore, the use of three antihypertensive agents would probably produce an unnecessarily large drop in BP in a proportion of "normotensive" recipients, with an associated significant incidence of hypotensive episodes. In the context of a population strategy, this combination may cause at least as much harm as good. However, whereas this proposed polypill has major shortcomings for use in the whole population, variations on this theme may have real potential benefits for use in the high-risk context. Several combination products are in development or production and it seems appropriate that their availability will should be greeted with enthusiasm by the increasing numbers who need to take several medications daily, and by those who prescribe them.

Combining Drug Therapies

The recently published ASCOT trial raised the fascinating possibility of an interaction between the statin atorvastatin and the two BP-lowering regimens (amlodipine and atenololbased). The effect of atorvastatin on coronary events when used in combination with these two BP-lowering regimens was significantly different. This appears to reflect an enhanced effect of the statin when used with the amlodipine-based regimen and a reduced effect when used with the atenolol-based regimen. Some data from other trials (e.g., the Prospective Pravastatin Pooling project) are consistent with these observations while others (e.g., the Heart Protection Study [HPS] and the Cholesterol Treatment Trialists' [CTT] Collaboration) are not. Nevertheless, interesting molecular biological studies are compatible with an interaction specifically between atorvastatin and amlodipine, and a hypothesis based on these studies has been generated to explain the apparent synergy on coronary events seen in the ASCOT Lipid-Lowering Arm (LLA) trial. Whether the effects of statins in general or atorvastatin in particular are genuinely attenuated by atenolol (or other β-blockers) requires further evaluation. Meanwhile, while it is possible that the interaction of BP- and lipid-lowering agents observed in ASCOT-LLA is a chance finding, any such interaction has exciting therapeutic significance.

Other Agents

Anticoagulants: Antiplatelet Agents and Antithrombotic Therapy

Coronary and Peripheral Atherosclerotic Disease

Aspirin 75 mg daily is recommended for life for all people with coronary or peripheral atherosclerotic disease. If aspirin is contraindicated, or there are side effects, then clopidogrel 75 mg daily is appropriate. Anticoagulation (e.g., warfarin with an international normalized ratio [INR] in the range of 2.0–3.0) should be considered for selected people at risk of systemic embolization from large MIs, heart failure, left ventricular aneurysm, or paroxysmal tachyarrhythmias.

Cerebral Atherosclerotic Disease (Non-Hemorrhagic)
For those with a history of cerebral infarction, or transient ischemic attack, and who are in sinus rhythm, aspirin 75–150 mg daily plus modified-release dipyridamole 200 mg twice daily is recommended for 2 years following the initial event to prevent stroke recurrence as well as other vascular events. If aspirin is contraindicated, or there are side effects, clopidogrel 75 mg daily is an alternative. For those who have a further ischemic cerebrovascular event while taking aspirin and modified-release dipyridamole, then changing aspirin for clopidogrel 75 mg daily should be considered.

Anticoagulation should also be considered for all people with atrial fibrillation who are at moderate (aged 60–75 years without additional risk factors) to high risk (>75 years, or >60 years with other risk factors such as hypertension, diabetes, or left ventricular dysfunction) to reduce the risk of a further stroke. If oral anticoagulation is contraindicated, or cannot be tolerated, antiplatelet therapy should be considered instead.

There is no evidence of benefit for anticoagulation in people with ischemic stroke who are in sinus rhythm.

High-Risk Individuals Without Established CVD
Aspirin 75 mg daily is recommended for all people over the age of 50 who have a total CVD risk ⩾20%, and in selected people with diabetes (>50 years, or who are younger but have had the disease for >10 years, or who are already receiving treatment for hypertension), once the BP has been controlled to at least the audit standard of SBP <150 mmHg and DBP <90 mmHg.

Agents that Reduce Blood Glucose Levels
Figure 3.17 provides a clear algorithm for when to intervene on varying degrees of IGF or IGT.

Glycemic Control in Diabetes
Good glycemic control has been shown in clinical trials to prevent micro-vascular complications in both type 1 and type 2 diabetes. In the UKPDS trial, people with type 2 diabetes with an average HbA1c of 7% (intensive treatment cohort) had considerably fewer microvascular complications than the conventional treatment cohort who had an HbA1c of 7.9%. This study also showed that good glycemic control had no beneficial effect on stroke

Fig. 3.17 Thresholds for intervention on glucose levels in asymptomatic people with CVD

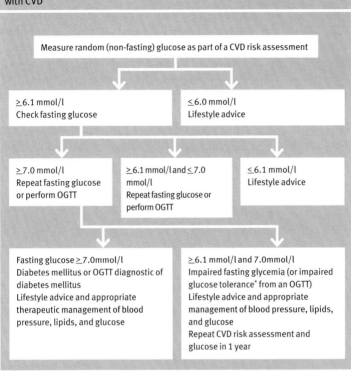

CVD, cardiovascular disease. *Impaired glucose tolerance: 2-hour glucose in an oral glucose tolerance test (OGTT) $\geq$ 7.8 mmol/l and $\leq$ 11.0 mmol/l. Reproduced with permission from the JBS 2 guidelines. *Heart* 2005; 91(Suppl 5):1–52.

but induced a favorable trend for a lower risk of MI (p=0.052). The Diabetes Control and Complications Trial (DCCT) showed clear evidence of benefit from good glycemic control in people with type 1 diabetes with respect to microvascular complications. However, this study was not sufficiently powered to give any information on macrovascular disease. Glycemic control is, therefore, important for people with either type 1 or type 2 diabetes. Ideally, the glucose target for type 1 and type 2 diabetes is normoglycemia (fasting glucose $\leq$6.0 mmol/l) with the avoidance of hypoglycemia and decompensated hyperglycemia. Optimal clinical management targets are a normal HbA1c level (<6.0%), and fasting or pre-prandial glucose values of 4.0–6.0 mmol/l. In clinical practice the practical HbA1c target is $\leq$6.5%, with an audit standard of $\leq$7.5%.

In type 1 diabetes, appropriate insulin therapy and concomitant professional dietary and lifestyle therapy are required for glucose control. In type 2 diabetes, professional dietary advice, weight reduction, and increased physical activity should be the first approach to achieve good glucose control. If these measures do not lead to a sufficient reduction of hyperglycemia, oral hypoglycemic drugs (biguanide, sulfonylurea, thiazolidinediones, or a combination of these) or insulin have to be added to the treatment regimen. Metformin is the drug of choice in overweight or obese people (BMI >25 kg/m^2).

Second-line agents could include sulfonylureas, post-prandial glucose regulators, and thiazolidinediones. An RCT of a thiazolidinedione in 5238 people with type 2 diabetes did not achieve the composite primary endpoint of all-cause mortality, non-fatal MI (including silent MI), stroke, acute coronary syndrome, coronary/leg revascularization, and leg amputation (HR 0.90, 95% CI 0.80–1.02). However, there was a reduction in the composite of all-cause mortality, non-fatal MI, and stroke (HR 0.84, 95% CI 0.72–0.98). Insulin treatment should be considered as soon as treatment with oral agents fails to achieve the audit target HbA1c of ≥7.5%.

The DIGAMI trials of people with an AMI and a glucose level ≥11.1 mmol/l evaluated a glucose insulin infusion followed by at least 3 months of insulin therapy. However, the second trial (DIGAMI 2) did not confirm the results of the first trial and there was no evidence of benefit in relation to total or coronary mortality or non-fatal CV events.

Chapter 4

Current Treatment Targets

Blood Pressure Targets

Most prospective observational data suggest that lower BP, lower the risk of adverse CV outcomes, although there has been some evidence suggesting a J-shaped relationship whereby the lowest levels of BP may be associated with increased CV morbidity or mortality. However, this may be a result of data misinterpretation brought about by "reversed causation"; for example, in certain circumstances low BP is the result rather than the cause of a pathological condition (i.e., heart failure) that is linked to an increased risk of morbidity and mortality. Similarly, chronic vascular damage in the capacitance vessels, which is linked to raised arterial pressure, is associated with falling DBP in elderly subjects. It is not surprising, therefore, that short-term follow-up of those with the lowest levels of DBP, in particular, will be associated with increased CV risk.

Data from RCTs has yet to answer the critical clinical question of how far BP should be lowered. However, best evidence to date has failed to demonstrate a target below which there is an apparent downside to lowering BP in terms of major CV events.

Although concerns have been raised in relation to BP lowering in those with established coronary disease, LVH or post-stroke, these concerns have not been validated by large morbidity/mortality trials. In a US trial, SHEP (Systolic Hypertension in the Elderly Program), DBP fell to 68 mmHg in the actively treated group. This reduction was associated with a significant decrease in CV events. In addition, many heart failure trials in which BP tends to start low or in which drugs are used to lower BP while treating heart failure (typically diuretics, β-blockers and ARBs or ACE inhibitors), have produced significant reductions in coronary events and death, providing further reassurance about effective BP lowering. As such, concerns about "overtreatment" and a "J-effect" appear to be largely misplaced.

There have been four trials designed to evaluate the extent to which BP should be lowered—the HOT trial, the UKPDS trial, the Appropriate Blood Pressure Control in Diabetes normotensive cohort (ABCD-NT), and the

N.R. Poulter, *Clinical Manual of Total Cardiovascular Risk*,
DOI 10.1007/978-1-84800-253-1_4, Springer-Verlag London Limited 2009

hypertensive cohort (ABCD-HT) trials. However, the latter three trials relate only to patients with diabetes. The results of these trials generally support a "lower the better" approach, but the results of the HOT trial, which have influenced recommendations on target BPs, failed to produce compelling evidence. This trial was designed to compare the effects of reaching three DBP targets: <90, <85, and <80 mmHg, but the BP range that was achieved was only 4 mmHg, rather than the 10 mmHg required by the study design. In addition, fewer than expected events occurred, and thus the study was underpowered to evaluate the original question using an ITT analysis. An optimal pressure of 139/83 mmHg was reported, but this used a less-than-ideal analysis of achieved BP effect. The data, as published, showed little advantage of lowering BP beyond 150/90 mmHg (see Fig. 4.1). In contrast, in the diabetic subgroup of the HOT trial, ITT analyses did confirm large significant reductions in total CV events in those randomized to reach <80 mmHg compared with those randomized to <90 mmHg (see Fig. 4.2), even though the actual achieved diastolic and systolic difference was about 4 mmHg. Further analyses suggest that among various subgroups of non-smokers, the lowest BP strata did enjoy significantly lower event rates, although these data require careful interpretation.

The data from the UKPDS and the two ABCD trials support the results found among patients with diabetes in the HOT trial that further BP lowering

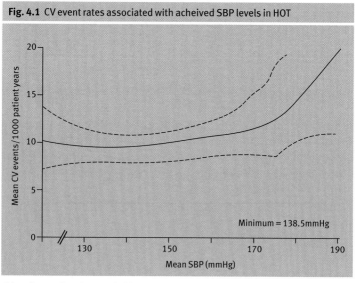

Fig. 4.1 CV event rates associated with acheived SBP levels in HOT

Minimum = 138.5mmHg

CV, cardiovascular; SBP, systolic blood pressure. *Dotted lines* indicate the estimated upper and lower values (95% CI). Reproduced with permission from Hansson L et al. *Lancet* 1998; 351:1755–1762.

Fig. 4.2 Significant benefits from intensive blood pressure reduction in diabetes (HOT trial)

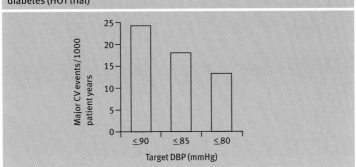

CV, cardiovascular; DBP, diastolic blood pressure; HOT, hypertension optimal treatment trial. Data from Hansson L et al. *Lancet* 1998; 351:1755–1762.

is advantageous. However, there is no compelling evidence in these trials for lowering SBP below 140 mmHg.

The Perindopril, pROtection aGainst REcurrent Stroke Study (PROGRESS), Heart Outcomes Prevention Evaluation (HOPE), and EUropean trial on Reduction Of cardiac events with Perindopril in stable coronary Artery disease (EUROPA) studies confirmed the benefits of additional BP lowering irrespective of baseline BP levels among patients with established vascular disease. Hence, the targets suggested by the HOT trial are likely to be too high in such high-risk patients. Finally, some of the benefits observed in the ALLHAT trial of a diuretic over both an ACE inhibitor and an α-blocker probably result from the better BP lowering achieved in the diuretic group. These benefits observed in ALLHAT were achieved in relation to mean SBP levels of 134 mmHg in association with allocation to a diuretic, compared with 136 mmHg associated with the other agents.

Current recommended targets from recent guidelines are shown in Table 4.1. It seems reasonable to accept that, as recommended by European guidelines, lower values than those recommended, if tolerated, are probably beneficial.

Summary
- There is a lack of robust trial evidence for optimal BP targets.
- Until such evidence is available, current BHS targets are the most evidence-based (HOT) and more logical (see Table 4.1).
- Targets should be lower for those with diabetes, renal impairment, or established vascular disease.

Table 4.1 BP targets in various recent guidelines

JNC 7	ESH–ESC	WHO–ISH	BHS 2004
‹140/90 mmHg	‹140/90*mmHg	SBP‹140 mmHg	‹140/85 mmHg
DM	DM	DM	DM
renal impairment	‹130/80	renal impairment	renal impairment
‹130/80		CVD	CVD
		‹130/80	‹130/80

BHS, British Hypertension Society; BP, blood pressure; CVD, cardiovascular disease; DM, type 2 diabetes; ESH, European Society of Hypertension; ESC, European Society of Cardiology; ISH, International Society of Hypertension; SBP, systolic blood pressure. WHO, World Health Organisation. *Lower if tolerated.

Lipid Targets

Cholesterol and LDL Cholesterol

No clinical trials have yet evaluated the relative and absolute benefits of cholesterol lowering to different pre-specified total and LDL cholesterol targets in relation to clinical events, although several trials have evaluated the "lower the better" hypothesis. Therefore, targets defined by guidelines are pragmatic and arise from the context of the total CVD risk of trial populations and, where available, pre-specified and post-hoc analyses of achieved total and LDL cholesterol concentrations.

The Prospective Pravastatin Pooling project reported significant relative reductions in all-cause and coronary mortality across most of the baseline LDL cholesterol concentrations from 5.5 mmol/l to 3.2 mmol/l. However, there was no significant treatment effect in the lowest quintile (<3.5 mmol/l) of the Cholesterol And Recurrent Events (CARE)/Long-term Intervention with Pravastatin in Ischemic Disease (LIPID) studies. Since then, in a trial by the HPS, a 1-mmol/l reduction in LDL cholesterol from 4.0 mmol/l to 3.0 mmol/l reduced the risk of major vascular events by about one-quarter, while reducing it from 3.0 mmol/l to 2.0 mmol/l produced the same relative reduction in risk. The evidence from this study has been reinforced by more recent statin studies (see Table 4.2). The Pravastatin or Atorvastatin Evaluation and Infection Trial (PROVE-IT), Treating to New Targets (TNT) and Incremental Decrease in End Points Through Aggressive Lipid Lowering (IDEAL) trials compared the effects of achieving different LDL cholesterol values by using either different statins or the same statin at different doses, but with no comparison placebo groups.

Table 4.2 Lipid-lowering treatment with a statin reduces the risk of CV events

Number of patients	Criteria	Treatment	Results
Anglo-Scandinavian Cardiac Outcomes Trial–Lipid-Lowering Arm (ASCOT-LLA)			
10,305	Well-treated hypertension	10 mg/day atorvastatin	Reduced the primary endpoint of non-fatal MI and fatal CHD by 36% (HR 0.64, 95% CI 0.50–0.83) by reducing LDL-C from 3.4 mmol/l to 2.3 mmol/l – a reduction of 1.1 mmol/l at 3 years compared to placebo
Collaborative Atorvastatin Diabetes Study (CARDS)			
2838	Type 2 diabetes, no history of CVD	10 mg/day atorvastatin	37% RR reduction (95% CI 0.48–0.83) in major CV events by reducing LDL from 3.0 mmol/l to 2.1 mmol/l
Pravastatin or Atorvastatin Evaluation and Infection Trial (PROVE-IT)			
4162	Recent acute coronary event	Intensive (80 mg/day atorvastatin) vs standard (40 mg/day pravastatin) statin therapy	16% RR reduction (95% CI 5–26%) from any cause or a major CV event (combined endpoint). This was achieved by reducing median LDL-C from 2.7 mmol/l at baseline to 1.6 mmol/l in the intensively treated group, compared to 2.5 mmol/l in the standard group
Treating to New Targets (TNT) study			
10,001	Coronary disease	80 mg/day atorvastatin vs 10 mg/day	With 80 mg, mean LDL-C values were reduced to 2.0 mmol/l, compared to 2.6 mmol/l with the 10 mg dose. This was associated with a RR reduction of 22% (95% CI 0.69–0.89) in new CVD events over a median 4.9 years. There was no difference in total mortality
Incremental decrease in endpoints through aggressive lipid lowering			
8888	History of AMI	80 mg atorvastatin vs 20/40 mg simvastatin	11% reduction in major coronary events (HR 0.89, 95% CI 0.78–1.01), which did not reach statistical significance. However, there was a 13% reduction in major CV events (HR 0.87, 95% CI 0.77–0.98). There was no difference in all-cause, CV or non-CV mortality

AMI, acute myocardial infarction; CHD, coronary heart disease; CI, confidence interval; CV, cardiovascular; CVD, cardiovascular disease; HR, hazard ration; LDL-C, low-density lipoprotein cholesterol; MI, myocardial infarction; RR, relative risk.

The primary endpoint was not significantly different in IDEAL, but a secondary endpoint, which included stroke and which matched the primary endpoint in TNT, showed a 13% (p=0.02) reduction. Similarly, when the primary endpoint in the PROVE trial (i.e., any CV event including revascularization) was considered in the IDEAL trial, there was an identical 16% risk reduction (p<0.0001). Furthermore, the primary endpoint results in IDEAL fit exactly on the regression line of the meta-analysis from the CTT collaboration. Therefore, the results of IDEAL are consistent with both PROVE-IT and TNT, and also with the meta-analysis from the CTT collaboration.

An intravascular ultrasound study of people with coronary disease (REVERSAL) also compared atorvastatin at doses of 80 mg and 10 mg but over a shorter duration. This study showed a significant reduction in progression of atherosclerosis in the intensively treated (80 mg daily) group, which was achieved by reducing LDL cholesterol from 3.9 mmol/l to 2.1 mmol/l.

The GREACE (GREek Atorvastatin and Coronary-heart-disease Evaluation) trial, which included people with coronary disease, compared managed ("treat to target") with usual care. To achieve the old NCEP ATP III target LDL cholesterol of <100 mg/dl (2.6 mmol/l), there was up-titration of atorvastatin in the managed-care arm. The NCEP LDL cholesterol goal was reached by 95% of the people in this arm (mean atorvastatin dose, 24 mg/day) compared to only 3% of the usual-care patients. In addition, total mortality (–43%), coronary mortality (–47%), coronary morbidity (–59% for MI and –52% for unstable angina), and stroke (–47%) were all significantly reduced. This was achieved by reducing LDL cholesterol from 4.7 mmol/l to 2.5 mmol/l in the managed-care group, providing a mean treatment difference of 1.9 mmol/l between managed and usual care.

The CTT collaboration reported an approximately linear relationship between the absolute reductions in LDL cholesterol achieved in these trials and the proportional reductions in the incidence of coronary and other major vascular events. The proportional reduction in the event rate per mmol/l reduction in LDL cholesterol was largely independent of the presenting level. Lowering the LDL cholesterol level from 4 mmol/l to 3 mmol/l reduced the risk of vascular events by about 23%, whereas lowering LDL cholesterol from 3 mmol/l to 2 mmol/l also reduced the residual risk by about 23%. Therefore, both individually and combined randomized trials support the view that in high-risk individuals any threshold below which lowering LDL cholesterol does not safely reduce CV risk is now at a much lower concentration—for example, <2.0 mmol/l for LDL cholesterol or <4.0 mmol/l for total cholesterol—than previously demonstrated. The NCEP ATP III guidelines were revised in 2004 and a lower LDL cholesterol target of <70 mg/dl (<1.8 mmol/l) is now advised for people at high risk.

Although the lipid target proposed in the 1998 JBS guidelines (i.e., a total cholesterol <5.0 mmol/l; LDL cholesterol <3.0 mmol/l) has now been superseded by new scientific evidence, it is still retained as an audit standard (see Table 4.3). This standard is consistent with the new General Medical Services (GMS) contract, which offers incentives for practitioners to achieve targets in the management of chronic disease, and applies to people with diabetes and those at high total risk of developing the disease. It represents the minimum standard of care for such high-risk people. Wherever possible, the optimal lipid targets of a total cholesterol of <4.0 mmol/l and a LDL cholesterol of <2.0 mmol/l, or a 25% reduction in total cholesterol and a 30% reduction in LDL cholesterol—whichever gets the person to the lowest absolute level—should be achieved.

Table 4.3 Optimal and audit standard lipid targets

CVD risk	Optimal total cholesterol target (mmol/l)	Audit standard for total cholesterol (mmol/l)	Optimal LDL cholesterol target (mmol/l)	Audit standard for LDL cholesterol (mmol/l)
Established atherosclerotic disease; CHD, stroke, or PAD	<4.0 or a 25% reduction in total cholesterol	<5.0	<2.0 or a 30% reduction in LDL cholesterol	<3.0
Diabetes mellitus	<4.0 or a 25% reduction in total cholesterol	<5.0	<2.0 or a 30% reduction in LDL cholesterol	<3.0
CVD risk >20% over 10 years	<4.0 or a 25% reduction in total cholesterol	<5.0	<2.0 or a 30% reduction in LDL cholesterol	<3.0

BP, blood pressure; CHD, coronary heart disease; CVD, cardiovascular disease; LDL, low-density lipoprotein; PAD, peripheral arterial disease. Reproduced with permission from the JBS 2 guidelines. *Heart* 2005; 91(Suppl 5):1–52.

Other Lipid Targets

There are no targets for HDL cholesterol and triglycerides, but an HDL cholesterol <1.0 mmol/l in men and <1.2 mmol/l in women and fasting triglycerides >1.7 mmol/l are each associated with an increased risk of CVD. In high-risk people with this pattern of dyslipidemia and in which this pattern persists after treatment with a statin has reduced LDL cholesterol below the target, additional therapy with a fibrate may be appropriate. The object of this additional treatment is to move toward the non-HDL cholesterol (total minus HDL cholesterol) and triglyceride values of <3.0 mmol/l and <1.7 mmol/l, respectively.

Glucose Targets

Ideally, the glucose target for type 1 and type 2 diabetes is normoglycemia (fasting glucose <6.0 mmol/l) with the avoidance of hypoglycemia and decompensated hyperglycemia. Optimal clinical management targets are a normal HbA1c (<6.0%), and fasting or pre-prandial glucose values of 4.0–6.0 mmol/l. In clinical practice the practical HbA1c target is <6.5%, with an audit standard of <7.5%.

It should be noted that there is no RCT evidence base for these recommendations but rather they are founded on strong epidemiological associations between increasing levels of glucose and/or HbA1c, and increasing rates of microvascular and macrovascular complications of diabetes. The results of, two major trials—ADVANCE (Action in Diabetes and Vascular disease: preterAx and DiamicroN modified-release Controlled Evaluation) and ACCORD (Action to Control Cardiovascular Risk in Diabetes)—have shown no clear cardiovascular advantages associated with lowering HbA1c levels in patients with type 2 diabetes (although renal benefits were apparent) and, indeed, ACCORD has given rise for concern about aggresive glucose lowering.

Chapter 5

The Doctor–Patient Relationship

Explaining Measures of Risk

There are various measures of risk in common usage (see Table 5.1). To briefly explain some of these measures, consider a population of 1000 people of whom 50 are exposed to a risk factor (e.g., smoking) and 950 are not (see Fig. 5.1). The crude absolute risk of an event over 10 years is 10% among smokers (5/50 × 100) and 2% among non-smokers (19/950 × 100). The relative risk of developing an event associated with the exposure is a fivefold increase compared with non-smoking (see Fig. 5.2); note, this has no units (they cancel out). Relative risk has no dimension of absolute risk — it merely informs how many more times the exposed is likely to suffer an event compared with the unexposed. However, the attributable or excess risk quantifies the extra risk (among the exposed) put "down to" the exposure.

Table 5.1 Measures of risk

Absolute	Population
Relative	Number needed to treat (NNT)
Attribute/excess	Global scores

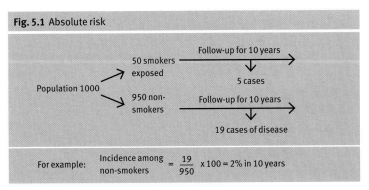

Fig. 5.1 Absolute risk

N.R. Poulter, *Clinical Manual of Total Cardiovascular Risk,*
DOI 10.1007/978-1-84800-253-1_5, Springer-Verlag London Limited 2009

65

Fig. 5.2 Relative and attributable risk

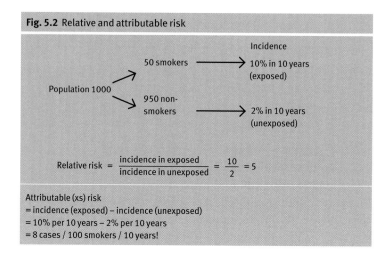

Relative risk $= \dfrac{\text{incidence in exposed}}{\text{incidence in unexposed}} = \dfrac{10}{2} = 5$

Attributable (xs) risk
= incidence (exposed) – incidence (unexposed)
= 10% per 10 years – 2% per 10 years
= 8 cases / 100 smokers / 10 years!

Hence, in the example shown, the attributable risk is eight "extra" cases per 100 smokers per 10 years.

From a population viewpoint, attributable risk is only useful if you know what proportion of your population are exposed (i.e., in the example shown—are smokers). If you know that, then the absolute number of extra cases can be calculated. This is known as PAR (see Fig. 5.3). In this example, the PAR is 4 cases/1000 population/10 years.

Thus, in this example, four of the five cases seen among the exposed are "down to" the exposure; one would have happened anyway as a background event rate (the 2% risk among non-smokers and hence of the total number of

Fig. 5.3 Population attributable risk

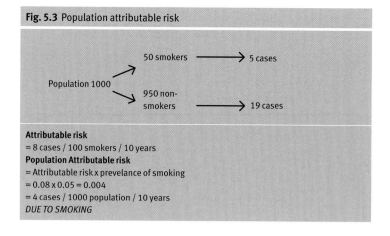

Attributable risk
= 8 cases / 100 smokers / 10 years
Population Attributable risk
= Attributable risk x prevelance of smoking
= 0.08 x 0.05 = 0.004
= 4 cases / 1000 population / 10 years
DUE TO SMOKING

24 cases [5 + 19]). Four would be prevented if the "exposure" was eliminated. This is the PAR fraction, which in the example shown is about 17% (4/24 × 100%).

The NNT in the example shown (if smoking were treatable and the risk reversible) would be calculated from the four cases per 50 smokers that smoking cessation would "prevent" (i.e., the attributable risk). If you "treated" all 50 smokers, four events would be saved and is calculated as 50/4 = 12.5 patients treated to save one event (NNT of 12.5 over 10 years). Global risk scores are discussed in Chapter 1.

Patient Compliance

Contemporary surveys from all over the world are consistent in showing that control of BP and lipid levels (as defined by being below currently recommended targets) is achieved only in a small minority of patients for whom current guidelines recommend treatment. Figure. 5.4 shows recent rates of treatment and control of BP and lipid lowering from various countries around the world. Possible explanations for the levels of control include:

- physician inertia;
- poor compliance;
- drug side effects;
- ineffective drugs;
- drug costs;
- guideline confusion;
- resistant hypertension or dyslipidemia.

Each of these possible explanations for poor control is likely to contribute to a variable degree. Rates of compliance or adherence and persistence with therapy have been reported in several settings and have been shown to be low. Non-randomized observational follow-up data suggest that after initiation of monotherapy with each of the standard antihypertensive agents, only a minority are still taking the therapy after 1 year. This lack of persistence can be explained by several reasons, including those listed above, and presumably a perception by the patient and/or doctor that continued treatment is not important.

Regarding BP-lowering efficacy and side effects, there is no doubt that individuals respond differently to different drug classes, and it is true that in a very small proportion of patients BP is resistant to therapy. In different healthcare settings the cost of BP- or lipid-lowering drugs is not acceptable to the patient and hence the patient may feel that any marginal benefits of treatment are not worth the cost. Similarly, it is easier and cheaper, at least

Fig. 5.4 Rates of BP control around the world

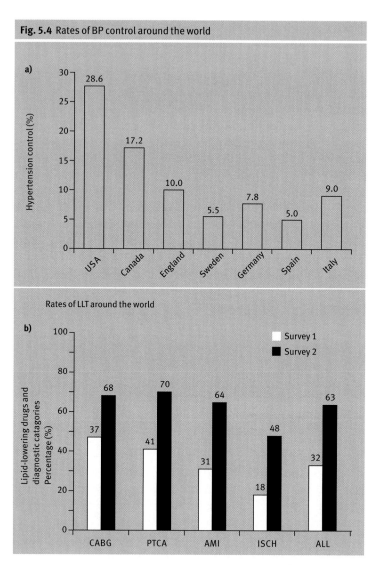

AMI, acute myocardial infarction; CABG, coronary artery bypass graft; ISCH, ischemia; PTCA, percutaneous transluminal coronary angioplasty. (**a**) Reproduced with permission from Wolf-Maier K et al. *Hypertension* 2004; 43:10–17. (**b**) Data from EUROASPIRE studies. *Eur Heart J* 1997; 18:1569–1582 and *Eur Heart J* 2001; 22:554–572.

short term, for the prescribing doctor not to bother to ensure careful follow-up of patients and their treatment.

Paradoxically, the production of guidelines on risk factor management can produce an adverse impact on best management. For example, in the context of hypertension, among the plethora of guidelines produced, there are potentially several (e.g., WHO–ISH, BHS, JNC 7, ESH–ESC) that might reach the general practitioner or hospital doctor. Historically, these guidelines have differed, causing confusion and frustration, which may in turn lead to inertia. However, even if the guidelines were consistent in all critical aspects, they all suffer from a common feature—length and complexity. This guarantees that they are not read and/or followed.

Whilst all the excuses listed above for poor control do tend to play a role in the majority of cases, the net result is not only inadequate control but also an intolerable burden of excess CV events. Among these excuses, perhaps the most important and remediable target for improving the status quo over BP and lipid levels is that of inertia on the part of the doctor. For example, it has been established that despite evidence of the need for at least two agents to achieve BP control, until as recently as 1998, 60% of patients on treatment for raised BP in England were only on one drug. A large European survey also showed that, when faced with patients not at BP targets (as determined by the doctor), 84% of such patients received a repeat prescription (see Fig. 5.5).

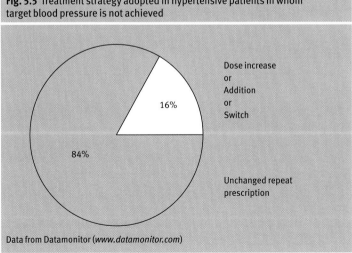

Fig. 5.5 Treatment strategy adopted in hypertensive patients in whom target blood pressure is not achieved

Dose increase
or
Addition
or
Switch

16%

84%

Unchanged repeat prescription

Data from Datamonitor (*www.datamonitor.com*)

In short, while genuine excuses for poor BP or lipid control may pertain to a minority of patients, most of these problems can be minimized by good clinical practice, as outlined in any of the major sets of guidelines.

For such an effect to be achieved, however, there needs to be major interventions by governments, in association with schools, the food industry, and through legislation. Meanwhile, the following actions could be undertaken by practicing doctors to improve compliance:

- ensure the patient understands the reasons and benefits of treatment;
- give clear instructions;
- repeat and reinforce instructions at each visit;
- inquire about side effects;
- put treatment regimes and objectives in writing;
- keep the treatment simple;
- use once-day dosing where possible;
- avoid mid-day dosing where possible;
- reinforce patient's participation in his/her own care;
- involve the patient's relatives, especially for the elderly patient; and
- involve the practice nurse in regular follow-up.

Establishing the Correct Regimen

Health policy treatment guidelines are, as far as possible, based on the best currently available evidence and ideally on RCT evidence. Inevitably, therefore, recommendations are usually made on the average patient included in these trials. How far the recommendations are applicable at the individual level remains variable and debatable. With increasing evidence, general treatment "rules" have become more flexible and tailored to individuals, such that thresholds and targets for interventions vary for different types of patients and the interventions themselves vary for different types of patients. However, in practice, optimizing interventions may be complex and difficult, due to frequently coexisting risk factors and co-morbidities. These complications have implications for compliance and adverse drug interactions become an increasing problem. For example, non-steroidal anti-inflammatory drugs and hypertensive agents, which are commonly used by elderly patients, interact to adversely affect BP control, whereas β-blockers and diuretics—particularly in combination—clearly adversely affect lipid profiles and glucose metabolism.

Consequently, the "art" of juggling with polypharmacy to generate optimal treatments across what may be several disease areas is an increasingly difficult problem. It is hard to see how this problem will be easily solved. While some variation of a polypill approach could reduce some of the problems within the CV area—for example, by combining lipid-, BP-, and glucose-lowering agents with an antiplatelet compound—the complexities of optimal dosing are enormous, and simplifying treatment regimens across disease areas appears impossible.

Ultimately, the target of disease prevention must be at the primordial level—that is, implementing non-drug lifestyle measures that could eliminate most of the chronic degenerative disorders that affect so many adults in an ever-ageing population. Simply treating established disorders such as hypertension, dyslipidemia, or dysglycemia with drugs is clearly not the best approach.

Chapter 6

Cardiovascular Disease Prevention: Prospects for the Future?

The ecological transition, whereby the major causes of death and disease in a population change with development, has a differential impact on different socio-economic strata within populations undergoing this process.

As populations develop, the burden of infectious diseases decreases in terms of morbidity and mortality and that of chronic degenerative diseases increases, in both absolute and relative terms. Consequently, it is predicted that the burden of CVD—primarily MI and stroke—will increase in relative and absolute terms over the next 10–15 years (see Fig. 6.1). This increase will take place in the face of our better understanding of the etiology of these disorders and of our having better means of treating the major risk factors that cause CVD and of treating CVD itself once established.

The reason for the anticipated increase in CVD is that most of the world is undergoing "development". On average, this process involves increasing longevity, body weight, alcohol, salt and fat intakes, and higher rates of smoking, while exercise and intakes of fruit and vegetables become reduced (see Table 1.8).

Within populations, the groups most affected by CVD differ, depending on the state of development of the population. For example, in the developed world, social class I (the professionals) are least affected by CVD, reflecting healthier diets and lifestyles. However, in the developing world, as CVD emerges—firstly with stroke and then CHD—it is in the professional classes that these disorders first appear. This reflects the earlier exposure of this socio-economic stratum to the adverse aspects of development. Over the ensuing one or two generations this inverse socio-economic gradient in CVD (highest rates in social class I) flattens out, eventually giving way to the direct association observed in the developed world (highest rates in the unskilled manual laborer).

N.R. Poulter, *Clinical Manual of Total Cardiovascular Risk*,
DOI 10.1007/978-1-84800-253-1_6, Springer-Verlag London Limited 2009

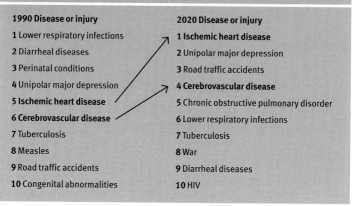

Fig. 6.1 Global burden of disease: change in rank order of disability* for the ten leading causes, 1990 and 2020

1990 Disease or injury	2020 Disease or injury
1 Lower respiratory infections	1 Ischemic heart disease
2 Diarrheal diseases	2 Unipolar major depression
3 Perinatal conditions	3 Road traffic accidents
4 Unipolar major depression	4 Cerebrovascular disease
5 Ischemic heart disease	5 Chronic obstructive pulmonary disorder
6 Cerebrovascular disease	6 Lower respiratory infections
7 Tuberculosis	7 Tuberculosis
8 Measles	8 War
9 Road traffic accidents	9 Diarrheal diseases
10 Congenital abnormalities	10 HIV

*As measured by disability-adjusted life years. Reproduced with permission from Lopez et al. *Nat Med* 1998; 4:1241–1243.

The determinants of these patterns of change are probably largely identified and hence the potential for genuine primordial prevention are huge.

Unless major environmental changes, which will pre-empt the anticipated lifestyle changes shown in Table 1.8, are introduced into the developing world as soon as possible, the currently massive burden of CVD will increase. Current high-risk treatment strategies will not be sufficient to offset these trends and only a concerted effort involving governments, the food industry, the media, the pharmaceutical industry, and the general population will prevent the anticipated global worsening of the current situation.

Suggested Reading

Chapter 1

Coronary Heart Disease Epidemiology: From Aetiology to Public Health, 2nd edition. Edited by M Marmot and P Elliot. Oxford: Oxford University Press, 2005.

Jackson R, Lawes CM, Bennett DA et al. Treatment with drugs to lower blood pressure and blood cholesterol based on an individual"s absolute cardiovascular risk. *Lancet* 2005; 365:434–441.

Lever AF, Brennan PJ. MRC trial of treatment in elderly hypertensives. *Clin Exp Hypertens* 1993; 15:941–952.

Wood D, Poulter NR, Williams B et al. JBS 2: Joint British Societies" guidelines on prevention of cardiovascular disease on clinical practice. *Heart* 2005; 91(Suppl 5): 1–52.

Yusuf S, Hawken S, Ounpuu S et al. Effect of potentially modifiable risk factors associated with myocardial infarction in 52 countries (the INTERHEART study): case-control study. *Lancet* 2004; 364:937–952.

Chapter 2

Alberti KG, Zimmet P, Shaw J; the IDF Epidemiology Task Force Consensus Group. The metabolic syndrome – a new worldwide definition. *Lancet* 2005: 366:1059–1062.

Alberti KG, Zimmet PZ. Definition, diagnosis and classification of diabetes mellitus and its complications. Part 1: diagnosis and classification of diabetes mellitus provisional report of a WHO consultation. *Diabet Med* 1998; 15:539–553.

Anderson KM, Wilson PW, Odell PM et al. An updated coronary risk profile: a statement for health professionals. *Circulation* 1991; 83:356–362.

Conroy RM, Pyörälä K, Fitzgerald AP et al. Estimation of ten-year risk of fatal cardiovascular disease in Europe: the SCORE project. *Eur J Hypertens* 2003; 24:987–1003.

Guidelines Sub-Committee. 1999 World Health Organization-International Society of Hypertension guidelines for the management of hypertension. *J Hypertens* 1999; 17:151–183.

Pocock SJ, McCormack V, Gueyffier F et al. A score for predicting risk of death from cardiovascular disease in adults with raised blood pressure, based on individual patient data from randomised controlled trials. *BMJ* 2001; 323:75–81.

Poulter NR. Measures of global risk: old versus new methods. *Clin Exp Hypertens* 2004; 26:653–662.

The sixth report of the Joint National Committee on prevention, detection, evaluation, and treatment of high blood pressure. *Arch Intern Med* 1997; 157:2413–2446.

Third Report of the NCEP Expert Panel on Detection, Evaluation, and Treatment of High Blood Cholesterol in Adults (Adult Treatment Panel III). *Circulation* 2002; 106:3143–3221.

Whitworth JA; World Health Organization, International Society of Hypertension Writing Group. 2003 World Health Organization (WHO)/International Society of Hypertension (ISH) statement on management of hypertension. *J Hypertens* 2003; 21:1983–1992.

Williams B, Poulter NR, Brown MJ et al. Guidelines for management of hypertension: report of the fourth working party of the British Hypertension Society 2004 – BHS IV. *J Human Hypertens* 2004; 18:139–185.

Wood D, Poulter NR, Williams B et al. JBS 2: Joint British Societies" guidelines on prevention of cardiovascular disease on clinical practice. *Heart* 2005; 91:(Suppl 5)1–52.

Chapter 3

ALLHAT Collaborative Research Group. Major outcomes in moderately hypercholesterolemic, hypertensive patients randomised to pravastatin vs usual care. *JAMA* 2002; 288:2998–3007.

ALLHAT Officers and Coordinators for the ALLHAT Collaborative Research Group. Major outcomes in high-risk hypertensive patients randomized to angiotensin-converting enzyme inhibitor or calcium channel blocker vs diuretic: The Antihypertensive and Lipid-Lowering Treatment to Prevent Heart Attack Trial (ALLHAT). *JAMA-Express* 2002; 288:2981–2997.

Amarenco P, Bogousslavsky J, Callahan A III et al.; ·Stroke Prevention by Aggressive Reduction in Cholesterol Levels (SPARCL) Investigators. High-dose atorvastatin after stroke or transient ischemic attack. *N Engl J Med*. 2006; 355:549–559.

Bloch MJ, Basile JN Treating hypertension in the oldest of the old reduces total mortality: results of the Hypertension in the Very Elderly Trial (HYVET) J Clin Hypartens: 10:501–503

Chobanian AV, Bakris GL, Black HR et al. Seventh report of the Joint National Committee on prevention, detection, evaluation, and treatment of high blood pressure. *Hypertension* 2003; 42:1206–1252.

Cholesterol Treatment Trialists" (CTT) collaborators. Efficacy and safety of cholesterol-lowering treatment: prospective meta-analysis of data from 90,056 participants in 14 randomised trials of statins. *Lancet* 2005; 366:1267–1278.

Dahlof B, Sever PS, Poulter NR et al; ASCOT Investigators. Prevention of cardiovascular events with an antihypertensive regimen of amlodipine adding perindopril as required versus atenolol adding bendroflumethiazide as required, in the Anglo-Scandinavian Cardiac Outcomes Trial-Blood Pressure Lowering Arm (ASCOT-BPLA): a multicentre randomised controlled trial. *Lancet* 2005; 366:895–906.

Dormandy JA, Charbonnel B, Eckland DJ et al; PROactive investigators. Secondary prevention of macrovascular events in patients with type 2 diabetes in the PROactive Study (PROspective pioglitAzone Clinical Trial In macroVascular Events): a randomised controlled trial. *Lancet* 2005; 366:1279–1289.

Guidelines Committee. 2003 European Society of Hypertension – European Society of Cardiology guidelines for the management of arterial hypertension. *J Hypertens* 2003; 21:1011–1053.

Hansson L, Zanchetti A, Carruthers SG et al. Effects of intensive blood-pressure lowering and low-dose aspirin in patients with hypertension: principal results of the Hypertension Optimal Treatment (HOT) randomised trial. HOT Study Group. *Lancet* 1998; 351:1755–1762.

Malmberg K, Ryden L, Wedel H et al; DIGAMI 2 Investigators. Intense metabolic control by means of insulin in patients with diabetes mellitus and acute myocardial infarction (DIGAMI 2): effects on mortality and morbidity. *Eur Heart J* 2005; 26:650–661.

NICE clinical guideline 34 (Partial update of NICE clinical guideline 18). Hypertension: management of hypertension in adults in primary care, June 2006. Available at: *www.nice.org.uk/page.aspx?o=CG034full guideline*. Last accessed November 2006.

Pedersen O, Gaede P. Intensified multifactorial intervention and cardiovascular outcome in type 2 diabetes: the Steno-2 study. *Metabolism* 2003; 52(8 Suppl 1):19–23.

Sacks FM, Svetkey LP, Vollmer WM et al; DASH-Sodium Collaborative Research Group. Effects on blood pressure of reduced dietary sodium and the Dietary Approaches to Stop Hypertension (DASH) diet. *N Engl J Med* 2001; 344:3.

Schwartz GG, Olsson AG, Ezekowitz MD et al; Myocardial Ischemia Reduction with Aggressive Cholesterol Lowering (MIRACL) Study Investigators. Effects of atorvastatin on early recurrent ischemic events in acute coronary syndromes: the MIRACL study: a randomized controlled trial. *JAMA* 2001; 285:1711–1718.

Scott R et al; Fenofibrate Intervention and Event Lowering in Diabetes (FIELD) Study: baseline characteristics and short-term effects of fenofibrate. Cardio vascular Diabetol 2005; 4:13.

Sever PS, Dahlof B, Poulter NR et al; for the ASCOT Investigators. Prevention of coronary and stroke events with atorvastatin in hypertensive patients who have average or lower-than-average cholesterol concentrations, in the Anglo-Scandinavian Cardiac Outcomes Trial – Lipid Lowering Arm (ASCOT LLA): a multicentre randomised controlled trial. *Lancet* 2003; 361:1149–1158.

The Diabetes Control and Complications Trial Research Group. The effect of intensive treatment of diabetes on the development and progression of long-term complications in insulin-dependent diabetes mellitus. *N Engl J Med* 1993; 329:977–986.

Third Report of the NCEP Expert Panel on Detection, Evaluation, and Treatment of High Blood Cholesterol in Adults (Adult Treatment Panel III). *Circulation* 2002; 106:3143–3221.

Turnbull F; the Blood Pressure Lowering Treatment Trialists" Collaboration. Effects of different blood-pressure-lowering regimens on major cardiovascular events: results of prospectively-designed overviews of randomised trials. *Lancet* 2003; 362:1527–1545.

UK Prospective Diabetes Study (UKPDS) Group. Intensive blood-glucose control with sulphonylureas or insulin compared with conventional treatment and risk of complications in patients with type 2 diabetes (UKPDS 33). *Lancet* 1998; 352:837–853.

UK Prospective Diabetes Study Group. Tight blood pressure control and risk of macrovascular and microvascular complications in type 2 diabetes: UKPDS 38. *BMJ* 1998; 317:703–713.

Wald NJ, Law MR. A strategy to reduce cardiovascular disease by more than 80%. *Br Med J* 2003; 326:1419–1424.

Williams B, Poulter NR, Brown MJ et al. Guidelines for management of hypertension: report of the fourth working party of the British Hypertension Society 2004 – BHS IV. *J Human Hypertens* 2004; 18:139–185.

Wood D, Poulter NR, Williams B et al. JBS 2: Joint British Societies" guidelines on prevention of cardiovascular disease on clinical practice. *Heart* 2005; 91(Suppl 5): 1–52.

Chapter 4

ALLHAT Officers and Coordinators for the ALLHAT Collaborative Research Group. Major outcomes in high-risk hypertensive patients randomized to angiotensin-converting enzyme inhibitor or calcium channel blocker vs diuretic: The Antihypertensive and Lipid-Lowering Treatment to Prevent Heart Attack Trial (ALLHAT). *JAMA-Express* 2002; 288:2981–2997.

Athyros V, Papageorgiou AA, Mercouris BR et al. Treatment with atorvastatin to the National Cholesterol Education Program goal versus "usual" care in secondary coronary heart disease prevention. The GREek Atorvastatin and Coronary-heart-disease Evaluation (GREACE) study. *Curr Med Res Opin* 2002; 18:220–228.

Cannon CP, Braunwald E, McCabe CH et al.; Pravastatin or Atorvastatin Evaluation and Infection Therapy-Thrombolysis in Myocardial Infarction 22 Investigators. Intensive versus moderate lipid lowering with statins after acute coronary syndromes. *N Engl J Med* 2004; 350:1495–1504.

Chobanian AV, Bakris GL, Black HR et al. Seventh report of the Joint National Committee on prevention, detection, evaluation, and treatment of high blood pressure. *Hypertension* 2003; 42:1206–1252.

Cholesterol Treatment Trialists" (CTT) collaborators. Efficacy and safety of cholesterol-lowering treatment: prospective meta-analysis of data from 90,056 participants in 14 randomised trials of statins. *Lancet* 2005; 366:1267–1278.

Colhoun HM, Betteridge DJ, Durrington PN et al; CARDS investigators. Primary prevention of cardiovascular disease with atorvastatin in type 2 diabetes in the Collaborative Atorvastatin Diabetes Study (CARDS): multicentre randomised placebo-controlled trial. *Lancet* 2004; 364:685–696.

Estacio RO, Jeffers BW, Hiatt WR et al. The effect of nisoldipine as compared with enalapril on cardiovascular outcomes in patients with non-insulin-dependent diabetes and hypertension. *N Engl J Med* 1998; 338:645–652.

Fox KM; EURopean Trial On reduction of cardiac events with Perindopril in stable coronary Artery disease Investigators. Efficacy of perindopril in reduction of cardiovascular events among patients with stable coronary artery disease: randomised, double-blind, placebo-controlled, multicentre trial (the EUROPA study). *Lancet* 2003; 362:782–788.

Grundy SM, Cleeman JI, Merz CN et al. Implications of recent clinical trials for the National Cholesterol Education Program Adult Treatment Panel III guidelines. *Circulation* 2004; 110:227–239.

Guidelines Committee. 2003 European Society of Hypertension – European Society of Cardiology guidelines for the management of arterial hypertension. *J Hypertens* 2003; 21:1011–1053.

Hansson L, Zanchetti A, Carruthers SG et al. Effects of intensive blood-pressure lowering and low-dose aspirin in patients with hypertension: principal results of the Hypertension Optimal Treatment (HOT) randomised trial. HOT Study Group. *Lancet* 1998: 351:1755–1762.

LaRosa JC, Grundy SM, Waters DD; for the Treating to New Targets (TNT) Investigators. Intensive lipid lowering with atorvastatin in patients with stable coronary disease. *N Engl J Med* 2005; 352:1425–1435.

Lewis SJ, Moye LA, Sacks FM et al. Effect of pravastatin on cardiovascular events in older people with myocardial infarction and cholesterol levels in the average range. Results of the cholesterol and recurrent events (CARE) trial. *Ann Intern Med* 1998; 129:681–689.

MacMahon M, Kirkpatrick C, Cummings CE et al. A pilot study with simvastatin and folic acid/vitamin B12 in preparation for the study of the effectiveness of additional reductions in cholesterol and homocysteine (SEARCH). *Nutr Metab Cardiovasc Dis* 2000; 10:195–203.

National Heart, Lung, and Blood Institute; National Institute of Diabetes and Digestive and Kidney Diseases; National Eye Institute; Centers for Disease Control and Prevention; National Institute on Aging. Action to Control Cardiovascular Risk in Diabetes (ACCORD) trial. Available at: *www.accordtrial.org/public/index.cfm*. Last accessed November 2006.

Nissen SE, Tuzcu EM, Schoenhagen P et al; for the REVERSAL Investigators. Effect of intensive compared with moderate lipid-lowering therapy on progression of coronary atherosclerosis: a randomised controlled trial. *JAMA* 2004; 291:1071–1080.

Pedersen TR, Faergeman O, Kastelein JJP et al. High-dose atorvastatin vs usual-dose simvastatin for secondary prevention after myocardial infarction. The IDEAL Study: a randomised controlled trial. *JAMA* 2005; 294:2437–2445.

PROGRESS Collaborative Study Group. Randomised trial of perindoprilbased blood pressure-lowering regimen among 6108 individuals with previous stroke or transient ischaemic attack. *Lancet* 2001; 358:1033–1041.

Schrier RW, Estacio RO, Esler A et al. Effects of aggressive blood pressure control in normotensive type 2 diabetic patients on albuminuria, retinopathy and strokes. *Kidney Int* 2002; 61:1086–1097.

Sever PS, Dahlof B, Poulter NR et al; for the ASCOT Investigators. Prevention of coronary and stroke events with atorvastatin in hypertensive patients who have average or lower-than-average cholesterol concentrations, in the Anglo-Scandinavian Cardiac Outcomes Trial–Lipid Lowering Arm (ASCOT LLA): a multicentre randomised controlled trial. *Lancet* 2003; 361:1149–1158.

SHEP Cooperative Research Group. Prevention of stroke by antihypertensive drug treatment in older persons with isolated systolic hypertension. Final results of the Systolic Hypertension in the Elderly Program (SHEP). *JAMA* 1991; 265:3255–3264.

Study rationale and design of ADVANCE. Action in Diabetes and Vascular disease – preterAx and diamicroN modified release Controlled Evaluation. *Diabetologia* 2001; 44:1118–1120.

The Heart Outcomes Prevention Evaluation Study Investigators. Effects of an angiotensin-converting–enzyme inhibitor, ramipril, on cardiovascular events in high-risk patients. *N Engl J Med* 2000; 342:145–153.

The Long-Term Intervention with Pravastatin in Ischaemic Disease (LIPID) Study Group. Prevention of cardiovascular events and death with pravastatin in people with coronary heart disease and a broad range of initial cholesterol levels. *N Engl J Med* 1998; 339:1349–1357.

UK Prospective Diabetes Study Group. Tight blood pressure control and risk of macrovascular and microvascular complications in Type 2 diabetes. UKPDS38. *BMJ* 1998; 317:703–713.

Waters DD, Guyton JR, Herrington DM et al. Treating to new targets (TNT) study: does lowering low-density lipoprotein cholesterol levels below currently recommended guidelines yield incremental clinical benefit? *Am J Cardiol* 2004; 93:154–158.

Whitworth JA; World Health Organization, International Society of Hypertension Writing Group. 2003 World Health Organization (WHO)/International Society of Hypertension (ISH) statement on management of hypertension. *J Hypertens* 2003; 21:1983–1992.

Williams B, Poulter NR, Brown MJ et al. Guidelines for management of hypertension: report of the fourth working party of the British Hypertension Society 2004 – BHS IV. *J Human Hypertens* 2004; 18:139–185.

Wood D, Poulter NR, Williams B et al. JBS 2: Joint British Societies" guidelines on prevention of cardiovascular disease on clinical practice. *Heart* 2005; 91(Suppl 5):1–52.

Chapter 5

Chobanian AV, Bakris GL, Black HR et al. Seventh report of the Joint National Committee on prevention, detection, evaluation, and treatment of high blood pressure. *Hypertension* 2003; 42:1206–1252.

Guidelines Committee. 2003 European Society of Hypertension – European Society of Cardiology guidelines for the management of arterial hypertension. *J Hypertens* 2003; 21:1011–1053.

Whitworth JA; World Health Organization, International Society of Hypertension Writing Group. 2003 World Health Organization (WHO)/International Society of Hypertension (ISH) statement on management of hypertension. *J Hypertens* 2003; 21:1983–1992.

Williams B, Poulter NR, Brown MJ et al. Guidelines for management of hypertension: report of the fourth working party of the British Hypertension Society 2004 – BHS IV. *J Human Hypertens* 2004; 18:139–185.

Chapter 6

Lopez AD, Murray CC. The global burden of disease, 1990–2020. *Nat Med* 1998; 4:1241–1243.

Index